NO GRAIN NO PAIN

Oskar Levsky

I dedicate this book to my son and all of you who suffer from pain and chronic inflammation. When your joints hurt so much that you cannot walk, when inflammation takes over your body, when ulcers bleed inside your stomach cavity, when no medicine brings relief, when physicians tell you there is no medical cure- don't give up hope. Suffering brings wisdom, strength and knowledge of the truth of life without grains and sugar.

In January of 2013, my son Max was diagnosed with an incurable chronic disease. Contrary to all of the doctor's expectations and medical prognosis that Max would be living in pain and have to take powerful prescription drugs for the rest of his life, Max completely recovered in six months by changing his diet and lifestyle.

This book is a personal testimony by the author and the information presented here cannot be used as medical advice, medical treatment, medical diagnostic tool or alternative therapy. Please consult a licensed medical practitioner prior to making any changes to your therapy, diet or lifestyle. The information presented here is not intended to replace a one-on-one relationship with a qualified health care professional. It is intended as a passing on of knowledge and information from personal research and personal experience. The author encourages you to make your own health care decisions based upon your research and always in partnership with licensed, trained and qualified health care professional.

If readers are taking prescription medications, they should consult with their physicians first and not take themselves off of medicines without proper supervision by qualified physicians. Medical treatments and medical errors are physician and patient responsibility. The author cannot be hold responsible.

CONTENTS

ACKNOWLEDGMENTS

My father and I were looking at the menu at a beautiful water-front restaurant in Greece and I could not make up my mind of what to order for dinner that night. The menu was written in Greek so I had no idea what it was saying. My father told me that day: "If you don't know what is good, then order what is expensive". We end up ordering grilled lamb chops and yogurt deep on the side called "tzatziki", a strained yogurt from goat milk, mixed with cucumbers, garlic, sea salt, olive oil and lemon juice.

Thirty years later, my twelve year old son was diagnosed with chronic, degenerative, inflammatory, autoimmune disease without a medical cure. What should I do, I asked my father over the phone? What should I give him?

Being an agricultural engineer since 1966 and being the head of the dairy industry for 7 years, my father had insider knowledge about food manufacturing practices, that were critical for Max's recovery against all odds and medical prognosis. As my father explained "the food we eat today is not the same food our ancestors use to eat." It is time to learn from our mistakes in order to protect our children and grandchildren.

INTRODUCTION

For the first time in US history, this generation of children in America may have a shorter life expectancy than their parents, according to a special report published in The New England Journal of Medicine, "the prevalence and severity of obesity is so great, especially in children, that the associated diseases and complications – Type 2 diabetes, heart disease, kidney failure, cancer – are likely to strike people at younger and younger ages". [1] Just two weeks later, I totally forgot about the report published in the most prestigious New England Journal of Medicine and in all major newspapers in the US. I went back to work as usual, never really anticipating the impact of the research findings or the consequences for my children. Few years later my twelve year old son became a statistic - diagnosed with chronic, inflammatory, degenerative, auto-immune disease, without a medical cure according to the Center for Disease Control and Prevention.

Sometimes too much health information in the media is rather confusing for most parents including myself. We are constantly bombarded with new information on a daily basis, so it is almost impossible to grab a hold of truth and use it against chronic inflammatory conditions of the brain, stomach, heart, liver, joints.

Most of the time there is no cure for these chronic diseases because they are not caused by germs, bacteria or viruses, but they are life style driven and can be avoided – they don't have to happen. For example, if you live in a small village on the northern island of Hokkaido and you cook farm fresh eggs in real butter for breakfast, wild salmon for lunch, grass fed beef, lamb or mutton for dinner, you will not have to worry about heart disease and diabetes striking your family. Real food will never hurt you. But if you work in Tokyo or Chicago and you live on comfort foods, crisp bread, bagels, coffee, donuts, pizza, pasta, honey nut cereal, hot-dogs, corn-dogs, breaded chicken, hamburgers, ketchup, mustard, corn chips, ice cream, cupcakes and caramel macchiato(s), then you should blame your boss for all that sugar, for being a pain in your neck and for causing you all that stress at work. The quick fix is always comfort food made with grain flour and sugar. Food companies know their business. They know all about you. Your fast paced, high stress, urban city lifestyle, plays very important role in developing addiction to sweet and comforting food. Why not? After all you've been working so hard, right? But, what excuse you have for poisoning your child with sugar? I had no excuse and I am very sorry.

The American Heart Association recommends not more than 100 calories a day from sugar if you are a woman and not more than 150 calories a day from sugar if you are a man. [2] Not more than 5% of all the calories in your diet should come from sugar. If you want to stay healthy, this is very important to remember, "Sugar comes into your body under 66 different names". Sugar is listed on the food labels as fructose, glucose, sucrose, table sugar, cane sugar, high fructose corn syrup, starch, malt, dextran, dextrin, agave syrup, treacle, panocha, lactose, sucanat, and 50 other names to choose from. Everything you eat is sugar coated, but all the blame goes to cholesterol, naturally produced by your liver. The cholesterol that is essential to life is not to be blamed for everything. There are over 80,000 commercially available foods on the market and about 75% of them contain added sweetener.

Many young parents in America like myself and many research scientists from around the world would like to know is a low fat, low cholesterol, whole grain diet sincerely good for my family? When carbohydrates such as grains enter your body, they are eventually broken down into glucose – blood sugar. We've been eating a low fat, low cholesterol, whole grain diet for the past 50 years in America. Today, we are sicker than any other nation in the world.

According to <u>OECD</u> Americans are currently spending $7960 per person, per year, on acute and chronic disease combined, totaling about $2.5 trillion dollars per year spent on health care. [3] The U.S. government is currently contributing 46% of the money or $1.13 trillion dollars per year in tax payers money for medical care, hospital beds and prescription drugs for the sick and disabled. There is no nation in the world that spends that kind of money on chronic diseases, hospital beds and prescription drugs. Recent studies show that <u>70 percent of Americans take prescription drugs</u>. [4]

How did this happen and why is it happening to our children?

"Americans spent $21.3 billion on cholesterol-lowering statin drugs in 2010 and the number of Americans taking statin drugs is set to double under the new guidelines unveiled by the American College of Cardiology and the American Heart Association. The goal is prescribing statins to as many as 70 million people". [5] How did this happen?

Too much health information in the media is rather confusing. Instead of adding to the confusion I want to share my personal testimony and research in a condensed format so that you can grab hold of the truth in 90 minutes and change your life. I will provide references on every subject so that you and your health care provider can extend your research when you have more time to find the answers to each question you might have. I am aware that this is a very difficult task to accomplish, but I believe the truth will save a nation.

Oskar Levsky is the founder and director of the Children's Environmental Health Agency and a consumer health advocate. He lives in Tokyo, Japan with his wife and two children.

Disclaimer: This book is a personal testimony by the author and the information presented here cannot be used as medical advice, a medical diagnostic tool or alternative medical therapy. Please consult a licensed medical practitioner prior to making any changes to your therapy, diet or lifestyle. The information presented here is not intended to replace a one-on-one relationship with a qualified health care professional. It is intended as a passing on of knowledge and information from personal research and personal experience. The author encourages you to make your own health care decisions based upon your research and always in partnership with licensed, trained and qualified health care professional.

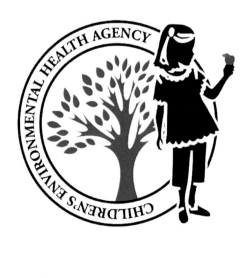

SKIN AND BONES

When I showed the prescriptions to the pharmacist, she looked at me with sorrow in her eyes. Who is this for, she asked me? It is for my 12 year old son, I responded with a shaky voice. I don't know why they prescribed him cancer medication when he does not have cancer. I was terribly confused and desperate. Max was waiting at home for the medicine. "Come back in one hour, the pharmacist told me. I will have the medicine ready for you by five".

I wished this was not happening, I wished it was just a nightmare. But once I arrived back home with my hands full with prescription drugs, I was reassured it was for real. My twelve year old son lost 30 lbs. in three weeks and looked miserable. The color of his skin was pale gray, he had excruciating abdominal pain, vomiting and suffering with diarrhea each hour. I found him on the couch curled up in a fetal position looking at me with his beautiful brown eyes that just few weeks ago were full with joy and now full with pain. He had no energy left in his weak body. My wife was sitting next to him. All we had in our hands to help our son was a big white paper bag filled with prescription drugs from the pharmacy and instructions explaining benefits, side effects and risks of taking these medicines.

"Medication Use: This medication is used with other drugs to treat a certain type of cancer (acute lymphocytic leukemia). It works by slowing or stopping the growth of cancer cells. Talk to your doctor about the risks and benefits, especially when used in children and young adults".

"Medication Side Effects: nausea, vomiting, diarrhea, and loss of appetite may occur. Temporary hair loss may also occur. Normal hair growth should return after treatment has ended. Remember that your doctor has prescribed this medication because he or she has judged that the benefit to you is greater than the risk of side effects".

4

How did all this happen? It seems like it happened overnight, but actually it took years for the disease to develop. Our kitchen was still hot from the thanksgiving dinner, vanilla cookies and sweet cinnamon apple pies baked every Sunday. We love to cook for our children and rarely eat out. Max loves home cooked food, but most of all he loves decadent chocolate chip cookies, syrup laden pancakes and sweet tea. He did eat his fair portion of cookies since he was a toddler.

We had just moved to California in hope of a fresh start, putting behind all the stress and financial hardship that we went through in Arizona during the worst housing crisis since the Great Depression that started back in October of 2007 after the leading US investment bank Lehman Brothers collapsed followed by the taxpayer bailout of City Group and Bank of America in January 2008. It was an experience we wish we never had to go through. Our beautiful home in Arizona lost 76% of its market value in less than six months. Millions in Arizona, Nevada and Florida, will remember the recession for the rest of their lives. I will never forget Christmas of 2007. The shopping mall in Scottsdale, where we had our store was completely empty. Six months into the recession and one in every three retailers in the mall was out of business. The customers vanished and foreclosures signs hung everywhere. There were entire neighborhoods of bank owned properties all over Phoenix.

We decided California would be our best option. We would leave Arizona behind and start a new life somewhere else. My wife secured a job in Los Angeles and I was hired in Beverly Hills by a startup luxury goods company. The luxury market in California was soaring. Fashion hungry customers from all over the world, but mostly from China were burning their extra cash buying expensive gifts, soft Italian leather shoes, French made designer coats, embellished sports cars and million dollar homes, all paid in cash. I had never seen that much cash in my life. No credit cards but crisp new dollar bills that looked and feel like they just came out of a printer. There were no signs of recession in Beverly Hills. Life was good again despite paying double the tax in California compared to Arizona.

We enrolled our children in the best school district. My daughter became a star on the high school basketball team. Max was playing baseball three times a week and also practicing water-polo. We were so glad to see our children happy again. Life was back to normal. We had new jobs, new home and new schools for our children. But, normal did not last long.

It was just before Christmas 2012, when we checked Max into the emergency room at the Children's Hospital Los Angeles. Max had an excruciating pain in his abdomen. During the next three weeks he lost over thirty pounds. I was able to count his ribs just by looking at them. He looked like a holocaust survivor, all skin and bones. We were paralyzed emotionally and exhausted physically in no time. Nobody in the medical community knew how to explain what happened to my twelve year old athlete who was in perfect health just few weeks ago? Crohn's disease was very bad news for Max because there is no medical cure. The pain and suffering can last for a lifetime. Inflammatory Bowel Disease (IBD) such as Crohn's, is one of the most painful degenerative inflammatory diseases that can manifest at any time in children and adults and it can last for a lifetime.

"IBD is one of the five most prevalent gastrointestinal diseases in the United States, with an overall health care cost of more than $1.7 billion. The two most common inflammatory bowel diseases are ulcerative colitis and Crohn's disease. This chronic condition is without a medical cure and commonly requires a lifetime of care. Each year in the United States, IBD accounts for more than 700,000 physician visits, 100,000 hospitalizations, and disability in 119,000 patients each year. Over the long term, up to 75% of patients with Crohn's disease and 25% of those with ulcerative colitis will require a surgery – Center for Disease Control and Prevention". [9]

"Sometimes ulcers can extend completely through the intestinal wall, creating a fistula — an abnormal connection between different parts of your intestine, between your intestine and skin, or between your intestine and another organ, such as the bladder or vagina. When internal fistulas develop, food may bypass areas of the bowel that are necessary for absorption. An external fistula can cause continuous drainage of bowel contents to your skin, and in some cases, a fistula may become infected and form an abscess, a problem that can be life-threatening if left untreated. Fistulas around the anal area (perianal) are the most common kind of fistula … In addition to inflammation and ulcers in the digestive tract, Crohn's disease can cause problems in other parts of the body, such as arthritis, inflammation of the eyes or skin, clubbing of the fingernails, kidney stones, gallstones and, occasionally, inflammation of the bile ducts. People with long-standing Crohn's disease also may develop osteoporosis, a condition that causes weak, brittle bones – Mayo Clinic". [10]

The Children's Hospital Los Angeles is one of the best hospitals in the U.S.A. The GI specialists working here are the best in the country. We are thankful for their sincere care. They did everything medically possible to help my son. Unfortunately, there is no medical cure for Crohn's disease. The options they have today at hospitals are limited to reducing the symptoms by medicating the child with antibiotics, painkillers, steroids, immune function suppressive drugs and powerful anti-inflammatory drugs, "this medicine is used to treat ulcerative colitis, a type of inflammatory bowel disease. It does not cure ulcerative colitis, but it *may* decrease symptoms such as diarrhea and rectal bleeding caused by irritation / swelling / inflammation in the colon / rectum. It is an amino salicylate anti-inflammatory drug. It is *believed* to work by keeping your body from making certain natural chemicals that *may* cause inflammation".

It sounds like a medical experiment, and in reality it is an ongoing experiment indeed. I just wish it was not my son they are experimenting on. The intentions were good, but unfortunately the options were limited to prescription drugs that did not bring any relief to Max's suffering. Surgery follows at some point and removal of the inflamed ulcerated portion of his colon is the only other option they have down the road for Max. However, after the surgery is over, it does not mean the child is now disease free. In Max's case of Crohn's disease the entire abdomen was affected with ulcers all over his digestive track including his stomach, duodenum, ileum, pan-colon, and rectum.

Max blood sedimentation rate (suggesting severe inflammation) was 20 times beyond the normal levels. Very soon he became anemic. He was losing his hair and he stopped growing too. The prognoses of living with Crohn's disease for the rest of his life was mind blowing and very scary with possible complications as the disease keeps progressing in the coming years.

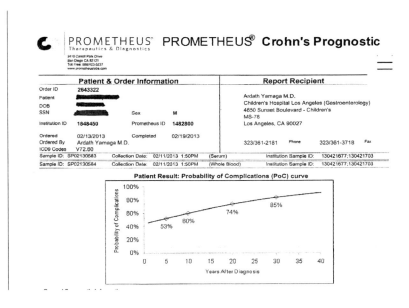

On the top of everything he developed arthritis symptoms with severe inflammation in the joints and could not move from excruciating pain in the hips, being unable to walk to the restroom on his own. Since he weighed about 70 lbs. at this point, I was able to carry him in my arms from the living room to the bathroom every 40-60 minutes. He was skin and bones and every move was painful. I was so afraid that if I was not nearby that he would probably try to walk on his own and break a bone.

We sent the fecal samples to The Mayo Clinic Medical Laboratories in North Carolina for analysis. The results were devastating. The Fecal Calprotectin Test (colon inflammation test) was showing 504 mcg/g. That was 28 times beyond the normal levels for a twelve year old child. Max's future with Crohn's disease did not look good.

Similar to a cardiovascular disease which starts as inflammation in the coronary arteries, Crohn's starts as inflammation in the gastrointestinal tract. Arthritis starts as inflammation in the joints. Alzheimer's disease starts as inflammation in the brain. From my own perspective, it does not matter what name they have for the disease when the symptoms are always the same: pain, inflammation and degeneration of human organs. They use the same or similar prescription drugs to treat these inflammatory conditions. In my personal opinion, if the symptoms are the same, then most likely the cause for these degenerative inflammatory conditions must be the same too.

"Is Max taking his medications?", my mother would ask me on the phone. Actually, she wanted to know if Max was doing any better. You see in today's world, taking your medication means getting better by masking the symptoms. Crohn's disease is incurable disease that can last for a lifetime. We desperately wanted Max to get better. Max was taking a variety of prescription drugs for the first 45 days, but he was not getting better.

Unfortunately his overall health condition was going from bad to worse day by day and sometimes by the hour. I decided to take time off from my job to be with my son. I was home in the morning and my wife was home in the evening. In just a short three weeks, Max's life was turned upside down. He could not walk on his own because of exhaustion and excruciating pain in the hips. He was not able to sleep any more from constantly running diarrhea. He was not able to digest anything because he would vomit after eating any food. He was not able to rest because of the excruciating pain in the abdomen. My son was suffering like no child should ever suffer and nobody was able to help him.

The insurance company called me and offered me free counseling for parents, to teach me how to cope with the new reality and preparing me for what is coming down the road. I refused the counseling and told them to remove my number from the call list. My son was going to be healed, I told them over the phone.

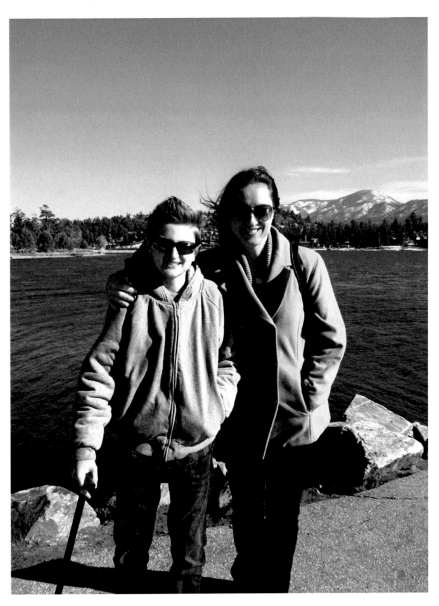

Just few weeks ago Max was swimming in the pool, playing water-polo and swinging the bat on the baseball field like a pro. How did this all happen? The medical prognosis was that he has to live with the disease for the rest of his life. Disabled and with Arthritis at the age of twelve? We received the blood test results from Prometheus, a San Diego based Therapeutic & Diagnostic Laboratories showing high probability for complications in a near future. The numbers were not good.

Tissue samples from his intestines (colonoscopy) were sent out to a different lab for more testing to assess the damage done to his gut. I am assuming they were looking for UFOs - unknown foreign organisms or maybe GMOs – genetically modified organisms. Regardless what kind of organisms they were looking for, the damage was already done, and according to the medical science there was no way back. He was sentenced to lifetime of suffering with inflammation, pain, ulcers, fistulas, and diarrhea.

Since the medical experts do not know the cause for this devastating degenerative disease, they blame it on the immune system claiming that Crohn's Disease is apparently an auto-immune disease.[11] This means the immune system is attacking tissues and organs in the body for no reason. This is a ridiculous and irresponsible medical speculation without solid scientific proof. Just because you cannot identify the cause for the disease, you should not classify the disease as an auto-immune disease and administer steroids and powerful drugs to suppress the child's immune system.

Max doctors were very smart and very careful. I am very thankful and very lucky to have the best specialists taking care of my son. You need solid evidence in medicine, not medical speculations. I can speculate because I am not a medical doctor who prescribes steroids and immune system suppressing drugs to children that are bleeding from the ulcers in the stomach. Being a physician is a very difficult job when there is no therapy nor medicine to treat the patient. It is a painful experience for the patient, and it is very frustrating for the physician. There is no medical cure for inflammatory bowel disease but there must be an underlying cause for the inflammation of the bowel.

 Instead of searching for a cure, searching for the cause made much more sense to me. Medical researchers are always focused on finding the cure and securing patent rights for the cure. I am not a medical research scientist looking for a pill to cure Crohn's disease. I am just a desperate father who loves his son. I decided to go the opposite direction and start looking for the cause of inflammation instead of looking for a cure.

If I could find and eliminate the cause, my son's immune system would do the rest. By eliminating the cause I was hoping to slow down the progression of the disease and give Max's immune system a chance to reboot and start working properly.

We are all created with an immune system able to fight germs, bacteria and viruses. But we are not well equipped to fight against man-made chemicals found inside our homes and chemicals find inside our food. [17]

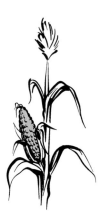

DOWNTOWN IN THE BREWERY DISTRICT

So how did we cure these chronic inflammatory degenerative diseases a hundred years ago? Well as a matter of fact, we did not have these horrific inflammatory diseases back in 1913. Diabetes, Coronary Heart Disease, Autism, Alzheimer's, Crohn's were not even mentioned in the medical school text books. Back in the day, our biggest health risks were lack of clean water and sanitation.

Not that long ago, our dairy cows use to eat grass, grazing outdoors on organic green pastures and producing the world's best quality milk and cream that was actually good for our children. Then something really bad happened, the small family farms quickly disappeared and the cows were confined in brick buildings downtown in the brewery district. Instead of grazing outdoors on green pastures, they were fed "steady diet of distillery slops leftovers from whiskey manufacture". [12] Confined in brick buildings without sanitation and clean water, the cows got very sick, the milk got contaminated with bacteria and mold and thousands of children died drinking tainted milk, "milk became an urban hazard". "The distilleries themselves owned some of the large herds of cows". After removing the cream, some milk dealers would add chalk dust, borax or plaster to give an appearance of whole milk". [12] Distillery slops or wet distilleries grains also called wet cake, represent the portion of the corn kernel that's left after the starch is removed and fermented for ethanol. Wet distilleries grains contain protein, fiber, fat, and about 35% moisture. It is fed primarily to cattle. The product has a shelf life of four or five days before it starts growing bacteria, mold, fungus and yeast.

Eating corn and distillery slops is not what cows were created for. They are herbivorous animals grazing on green pastures. "Cows grazing on pasture and receiving no supplemental feed, had 500% more conjugated linoleic acid (CLA) in their milk fat compared to cows fed typical dairy diets". [13]

After the war, (1939-1945) thanks to advances in science and technology everything changed again, for better or for worse. We became consumers of technologically advanced processed foods: multigrain breakfast cereals, pasteurized milk with an extended shelf life, bleached wheat flour products, processed meats loaded with nitrates, hot dogs, burgers, and sloppy joes surrounded by a fluffy white bun, pizza, french fries, potato chips, soda-pop, corn starch, corn chips, corn oil, and corn syrup based beverages, plus hundreds of sugar packed candy bars and granola bars to choose from. We are talking mostly grains, sugar, starch, and hydrogenated vegetable oils. Manufacturing food is not the same as growing food.

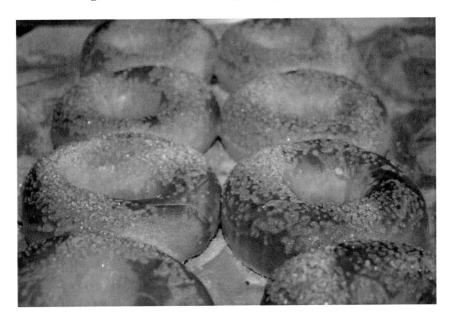

The food manufacturers today are using a variety of food additives and preservatives into their manufacturing formulas. Many of these food additives and preservatives are powerful chemicals you should not be playing with in your kitchen. For better illustration, let's have a look at the ingredients of the most popular food in America.

Here is the list of the 50+ ingredients in the original sugar glazed donut. Please do not mix these food ingredients at home, unless you have a degree in bio-chemistry from The Harvard School of Public Health.

Ingredients: Enriched bleached wheat flour (contains bleached wheat flour, niacin, reduced iron, thiamine mononitrate, riboflavin, folic acid), dextrose, vegetable shortening (partially hydrogenated soybean and/or cottonseed oil), water, sugar, soy flour, egg yolks, vital wheat gluten, yeast, nonfat milk, yeast nutrients (calcium sulfate, ammonium sulfate), dough conditioners (calcium dioxide, monocalcium and dicalcium phosphate, diammonium phosphate, sodium stearoyl-2-lactylate, whey, starch, ascorbic acid, sodium bicarbonate, calcium carbonate), salt, mono- and diglycerides, ethoxylated mono-and diglycerides, lecithin, calcium propionate (preservative), cellulose gum, malted barley flour, natural and artificial flavors, enzymes, sodium caseinate, corn maltodextrin, corn syrup solids and BHT (to help protect flavor). **Glaze contains:** Sugar, water, corn starch, calcium carbonate, calcium sulfate, agar, dextrose, locust bean gum, disodium phosphate, sorbitan monostearate, mono-and diglycerides, artificial flavor and salt. [14]

Thanks to today's cutting edge science and technology, our children eat processed foods every day instead of real farm fresh food our grandfathers use to eat. Before the war, our burgers use to have only one ingredient – grass fed beef. Today, the burgers served in the public schools across America have an amazing 26 ingredients according to the resent report by NPR's Allison Aubrey. "What is inside the 26-ingredient school lunch burger ". [15]

Are you still wondering why this generation is obese and suffering at a very young age with A variety of degenerative and inflammatory diseases? These are life style driven disease and can be avoided and sometimes even reversed. Most of the time it is not in the genes of our children to get sick, but it is in the food ingredients they eat every day. The food our children eat today is highly processed, altered, genetically modified and sometimes even contaminated with toxic chemicals.[17] The child's immune system will react with allergies and inflammation in different organs including the brain, leading to behavioral and learning disabilities.

On the other side, a child's digestive system is chronically overloaded with sugar, grains, gluten, starches, and high fructose corn syrup find in processed foods and beverages. The elevated blood sugar often binds to the proteins creating toxic bonds known as AGEs [18] that further can cause free radical damage and inflammation throughout the child's body and brain. This is overwhelming for the child's immune system to function properly. The stage is now set for chronic inflammatory diseases.

You should know what is pure, natural and good for you. You can drink factory processed genetically modified soy milk as much as you want, but you will never receive the health benefits of drinking grass fed goat milk from your own farm. There is no replacement for grass-fed beef regardless how much grass, wheat, and oats you eat every day. My son has consumed twice more grass, wheat and oats from grain cereals and granola bars during his first 12 years of life than my father consumed in 73 years. I have never seen my father eat breakfast cereal with sugar and milk. My father has never had a bowl of cereal period. He loves salmon, shrimp, champagne, watermelon and strawberries for breakfast.

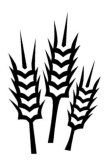

Dwight Lundell, M.D., world renowned heart surgeon, speaks out on what really causes inflammation and heart disease: "We physicians with all our training, knowledge and authority, we often acquire a rather large ego that tends to make it difficult to admit we are wrong. As a heart surgeon with 25 years of experience, having performed over 5,000 open-heart surgeries, today is my day to right the wrong with medical and scientific facts". Dr. Lundell is the past Chief of Staff and Chief of Surgery at Banner Heart Hospital in Mesa, Arizona. He is the author of the best-selling book "The Cure for Heart Disease [19] http://amzn.com/0979034000

In 2010, the Office of Inspector General for the Department of Health and Human Services said that bad hospital care contributed to the deaths of 180,000 patients in Medicare alone in a given year. The Journal of Patient Safety says the numbers may be much higher – between 210,000 and 440,000 patients each year who go to the hospital for care suffer some type of preventable harm that contributes to their death. That would make medical errors in hospitals – the third-leading cause of death in America, behind heart disease, which is the first, and caner, which is second leading cause of death [20] (NPR NEWS, How Many Die From Medical Mistakes In U.S. Hospitals? - by Marshall Allen 09/20/2013)

CUTTING EDGE FOOD SCIENCE

Would you consider genetically modified corn be categorized as food? Would your stomach enjoy the glyphosate found in genetically modified grains and beans. Would your intestinal bacteria continue to live or die in the presence of glyphosate?

The food industry made it legal to sell genetically modified organisms in the USA without labels. The tax payers being ignorant and miss-informed, they voted against labels for genetically modified food.

Russia's Federal Agency for Agricultural Control officially banned all GMO corn imports in 2012 in response to the very alarming study conducted in France, that found rats developed <u>horrifying tumors all over their bodies</u> and in their internal organs when they were fed genetically modified corn. [21] If I knew that the tortilla chips we had been eating for years were made with genetically modified corn, if there was a label on the box, I would have never bought the corn chips to begin with. I simply did not know what is inside the box. I did not know that this genetically modified corn has glyphosate that can interrupt the metabolic functions of the intestinal bacteria, bypassing and destroying Max's immune system barriers and exposing him to dangerous toxins that will cause severe destruction and inflammation all over his body as explained by <u>Dr. Stephanie Seneff, PhD</u> in her latest research paper, published on April 18th 2013 in *Entropy*, Volume 15, Issue 4, Pages 1416-1463. [7]

Ten years ago my wife enrolled in a PhD program in natural health and since then we built an entire library in our home. I went through all the books in less than two months. I dedicated all of my time to find the cause for Max's devastating Crohn's disease. I learned that it is illegal in the US to use the word "natural medicine" because only the federal food and drug administration can grant you permission to call "the cure", cure and to call "the medicine", medicine. The entire world from Greece to Japan has been using food as a medicine for thousands of years, but not America. Maybe that is good since real food requires no doctor's prescription, at least not yet. Make sure you go out to vote the next time we have elections. Check all the propositions on your ballot and cast your vote for mandatory GM food labels and labels for foods with added sugar. Your health and your future depend on your vote.

The ancient Greek physician Hippocrates (460 BC – 370 BC) who is considered the father of western medicine, wrote: "Let food be thy medicine and medicine be thy food" [22.] Hippocrates endured a 20-year prison sentence during which he wrote well known medical works such as *The Complicated Body*, encompassing many of the things we know to be true today. The Hippocratic Oath for physicians is still relevant and in use today in the USA.

Today we know that nutrients are molecules that provide nourishment essential for growth and maintenance of life. Their job is to nourish, repair, restore, and rebuild our cells, tissues and organs.

The word "restaurant" literary means "food that restores", food that will bring back a person's strength. The first shop of this kind opened in Paris in 1765 and was serving "bouillons restaurants", meat based consommés intended "to restore a person's strength". Ever since the Middle Ages the word restaurant had been used to describe any of a variety or rich bouillons made with chicken, beef, onions, herbs.

The average age of the cells in an adult's body is about seven. Every cell in your body is replaced with a new one every seven to ten years if the building blocks called nutrients are available. We call these life supporting elements "essential minerals" and we get them from the earth's rich soil, calcium, magnesium, sodium, potassium, sulfur, phosphorus, chloride as well as "trace minerals" such as iron, zinc, iodine, selenium, copper, manganese, fluoride, chromium, molybdenum. Besides essential minerals and trace minerals, we need vitamins: amino acids, proteins, enzymes, carbohydrates and fats to stay alive. Each one of these nutrients is important for the life functions inside your cells, so that your cells, tissues, and organs, can function properly. Every time that you are deficient in some nutrient, you will experience some sort of functional disability on a cellular level. The body will try to fix the problem by replacing the missing element whenever possible. Unfortunately food is the last thing you will study in medical school.

As you already know from your high school biology class, we are made up of 80% water and 20% minerals such as calcium, magnesium, sodium, potassium, sulfur, phosphorus, chloride. According to modern day science, we are made of water and mineral dust just like is described in the book of Genesis 2:7 - "And the Lord God formed man of the dust of the earth" .

Nutrients are life supporting molecules that provide nourishment essential for growth and the maintenance of life. On the other side, the lack of nutrients in your food and the presence of chemicals in your environment such as heavy metals, lead, mercury, asbestos, volatile organic compounds, pesticides, herbicides, fungicides, ammonia and formaldehyde can cause a serious damage to your cells, tissues and organs, turning normal living cells into cancer cells. It usually takes months and years for these carcinogens to build up and to cause cancer in humans. The cause for chronic disease is always the same too many toxins and too little nutrition. The human body is actually very resilient and able to eliminate toxins and even cancer cells efficiently. However "the chemical body burden sometimes is too big for your immune system to cope with the toxic overload" [23.] - Dr. Daniel Rubin, ND

So what happens next in the human body after cancer sets in is a huge chaos of events. The cancer cells will multiply very fast through fermentation in the sugar rich body environment. The sugar acts like a fuel for cancer growth. That's why all the people that have been diagnosed with cancer are craving sugar, bread, coffee, donuts, cookies, sweets, candies, chocolate, ice-cream. The excessive consumption of refined sugar contributes to the acidic body environment, needed for cancer growth. The saliva PH test in people with cancer is always acidic. You can test your saliva at home. All you need is PH testing tape that you can buy at your local pharmacy. "Cancer can only grow in a sugar rich acidic body environment, and multiply through fermentation". [24] - Sir. Arnold Takemoto

The sugar rich acidic body environment is also a perfect feeding ground for microorganisms such as bacteria, mold, fungus and yeast. These living organisms feed on sugar and they produce toxins and mycotoxins as waste product that can cause all kinds of health problems in humans but also in farm animals, especially in dairy cows that eat stored animal feed (grains). "Mycotoxins can appear in the food chain as a result of fungal infection of the crops, either by being eaten directly by humans or by being used as livestock feed. Mycotoxins greatly resist decomposition or being broken down in digestion, so they remain in the food chain in meat and dairy products. Even temperature treatments, such as cooking and freezing do not destroy some mycotoxins". [25]

Coffee, donuts, refined sugar and grain cereals are perfect combination for creating a sugar rich acidic body environment. By eating processed foods made with grain flour and sugar your immune system never gets a break. Instead of dealing with the disease, your immune system is busy with digestion and breaking down gluten, starches, grains, sugar and dealing with pathogenic bacteria, mold, fungus, and yeast that feeds on sugar and grains. Did you know that your gut is the most important part of your most complex and sophisticated immune system? Your intestines are immune system barriers – your first line of defense against bacteria, toxins, mold and fungi yeast . When your gut is not functioning properly, you don't have immunity to anything. Give your gut a break by completely eliminating sugar, grains and starchy foods from your diet. Give your immune system a chance to reset, reboot and start working efficiently, for maybe the first time in your life. "The brain is not the only place in the body that's full of neurotransmitters. A hundred million neurotransmitters line the length of the gut, approximately the same number that is find in the brain" [26.] "Your gut is your second brain" - <u>Dr. Michael Gerson</u>

Have in mind that going on a sugar fast is very difficult and very few people have done an extensive sugar detox program. However, it is the only way to clean your digestive system from the pathogenic microorganisms that live in your intestines and feed on sugar 24/7. The cravings for sugar are so strong that nine out of ten people will keep eating sugar and grains regardless of the consequences to their health. It is very difficult because their intestinal bio-flora is very different. People that are on a high sugar diet have a different kind of bacterial colonies in their gut compared to the people that eat mostly grass-fed lamb as in New Zealand, raw fish as in Japan, and fresh fruits and vegetables as in Greece. Picture your stomach for a moment and billions of sugar digesting bacteria, fungi and yeast covering every square inch of your gut and asking for more sugar 24/7. That is why is so difficult to quit sugar, bread, pasta, coffee, donuts, grain cereals. For Max, the pain, the ulcers, the diarrhea, the suffering was so unbearable that he had no choice but to quit the consumption of sugar and grains completely.

After fasting from sugar, starches and grain for forty days, all the sugar feeding bacteria in his intestines, all the fungi, mold and yeast died off from starvation. Max claimed back his health, and so can you. You must talk to you doctor before starting any therapy, diet or fast. This is very important because without sugar you are going to feel very sick at the beginning and even more sick later when all that bacteria dies off inside your intestines and all the toxins are getting expelled out of your body through the kidneys. Your doctor needs to make sure that your kidneys are healthy to do the job. Imagine all the toxins leaving your body at once. Forty days after starting your sugar fast, you are going to feel great. You are going to feel like a new person. The sugar fast is going to have positive impact on every cell and every organ in your body.

I was 30 years old when I had my very first spoonful of grain cereal. Back in February of 1997 when I first arrived in America I was given a breakfast cereal with milk. I did not know what was in it nor did I know how to eat it. They gave me a spoon. I had never tried anything like this having been in Macedonia my entire life. It tasted like shredded cardboard coated with sugar. I know that sounds like nonsense to you, but I have never had cereal in my life. My son, on the contrary, had his first spoonful of cereal when he was about 11 months old and he continued eating many different kinds of cereals for the next 11 years, until the day he was diagnosed with inflammatory Crohn's Disease. I was desperate to help my son. Searching for answers, I asked the doctors at the children hospital how it happened and what was the cause? Maybe it was the tortilla chips he was enjoying every day after school, or maybe the variety of gluten-free cereals for breakfast. Was the cause for the inflammation hidden in the genetically modified corn chips, or the breakfast cereals loaded with sugar?

The answer to my question was that "no food can do damage like that". Crohn's Disease is most likely an auto-immune disease, they explained to me, "we don't know what the cause is for the inflammation or the stomach ulcers, but we cannot blame it on any particular food". I respectfully disagree. The truth is that if the medical doctors didn't follow the protocols, they risked their reputation. Medicine is a business; the physicians must follow the established protocols to get paid by the insurance company. On the other side, I get paid nothing from your insurance companies by sharing the truth with you. I know that real food is critical for your health and well-being. I know that the old world cuisine of my grandmother is the absolute best choice when it comes to inflammation and nourishing a sick person back to health. It can actually change your life or maybe even save your life. Farm fresh food, not changed, not modified, not processed-food is good for you. Visit local farms, get to know the farmers, and treat your grass fed beef and butter as real food, just like the Jews and the Greeks did for the past 6000 years.

Today 88 % of the U.S. corn, 94 % of soybeans, 90 % of cotton (cottonseed oil is in thousands of food products), 90 % of canola, and 95 % of sugar beets are genetically engineered [27.] Many of these major crops enter packaged foods in various forms. It is estimated that 80% of the processed foods on supermarket shelves contain genetically modified organisms.

Max tried many different medications looking for the one that actually works. The five groups of drugs used to treat Crohn's Disease today are aminosalicylates (5-ASA), steroids, immune modifiers (azathioprine, 6-MP, and methotrexate), antibiotics (metronidazole, ampicillin, ciprofloxin, others), and biologic therapy (inflixamab). Keep in mind that none of these powerful prescription drugs deals with the disease directly because the cause is unknown. Masking the symptoms instead of dealing with the disease directly was the only option we had at the time.

Hoping for better outcome, Max had no choice but to follow the medical protocol we were offered. On the other side, I knew that the cure is always in the cause, not in the prescription drugs. I knew that if I could just identify the cause, my son would be saved from the pain and suffering. However, I needed time that I did not have. I was not a scientist playing in a lab doing a medical research on chronic diseases. I was not experimenting with different drugs on mice in my laboratory. It was my own son they were experimenting on with different processed foods since the day he was born and now with different prescription drugs along with horrifying side effects.

The scientific data and many medical research papers published in Germany in the past three years point to gluten, grains, and sugar in processed foods as the leading factor in the development and progression of inflammatory chronic conditions, [28] degeneration of organs [29] and premature aging. [30]

A new research paper was published in France that has shaken the world from Paris to Tokyo. "Eating genetically modified corn and consuming trace levels of Monsanto's roundup chemical fertilizer caused rats to develop horrifying tumors, widespread organ damage, and premature death. That's the conclusion of a shocking new study [31] that looked at the long-term effects of consuming Monsanto's genetically modified corn." "I am shocked by the extreme negative health impacts" says Dr. Michael Antoniou, molecular biologist, King's College London. "We can expect that the consumption of GM maize and the herbicide Roundup, impacts seriously on human health."

According to Jeffrey Smith with the Institute of Responsible Technology we are gambling with our lives [32] In my personal opinion, if the genetically modified corn can cause laboratory animals to develop these horrifying tumors, what are the effects on our cattle?

The only human feeding study on GMOs ever conducted showed that genes "jumped" from GM soy into the DNA of human intestinal bacteria and continued to function. That means that long after you stop eating GM soy, you may still have GM proteins produced continuously inside of you. What if the pesticide-producing "Bt" gene found in GM corn chips were also to jump? It might transform our intestinal flora into living pesticide factories, and possibly for the long term [33.]

Max was given powerful antibiotics. However there were no pathogenic bacteria found in his intestines. There was no bacterial infection. Why are they giving him medicine that makes him sicker? Why is he losing weight so rapidly? Why are they giving him medicine for cancer? Is he at risk for developing cancer? Why does the diarrhea never stop? Too many unknowns and too much information was not really helping me to narrow down my search for health and a possible recovery for my son. We had done all the tests available at the children's hospital, blood, urine, and fecal analysis, including a colonoscopy and endoscopy with a small camera traveling through the stomach, through the small and large intestines and then out. We could see the ulcers and the inflammation by taking pictures of the gastrointestinal track. However, all the blood work and the biopsy tests came in negative for pathogenic bacteria or even infection. The ulcers were everywhere, and the inflammation in his colon measured by the fecal calprotectin inflammation marker was twenty eight times above the normal levels.

I was told that the genetically modified corn chips and the high fructose corn syrup had nothing to do with my son's disease, the stomach ulcers, the inflammation, the constant diarrhea. No food can do that kind of damage, I was told over and over. On the flip side, Dr Michael Antoniou molecular biologist at The King's College London said just few months ago, "We can expect that the consumption of GM corn will have serious impact on human health" [34.] Dr. Michael Antoniou blew the whistle in 2012 and Dr. Stephanie Seneff, Ph.D. [35] confirms the toxicity of glyphosate in 2013 in her latest research paper published 4/18/2013 – watch video.

Dr. Stephanie Seneff dedicated 30 years of her life to research, to put all the scientific data together, to uncover the truth buried in American soil by American scientists playing farmers. I believe the truth will save a nation, or at least this generation.

Playing "genetic roulette" with our children is morally wrong and catastrophic. In twenty years from today one in every two children in America will be diagnosed with inflammatory or autoimmune disease before they turn twelve.

<u>Breaking News</u> by Reuters, May 5th, 2014 "French ban on GMO maize cultivation gets final approval".

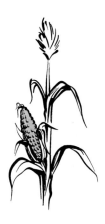

FATHER'S DAY CONFESSION

I had to find answers quickly; we were running out of time. I was committed to finding the cause, knowing that the cure is always hidden in the cause. I was shocked once I realized that the cause was right in front of me, hidden in the processed foods loaded with sugar, grains, and refined vegetable oils. The cause for inflammation was hidden in the breakfast cereals, the corn chips, the soda pop, the granola bars, the sweet tea. Reality hit me hard. I was responsible for the disease. It was I buying cheap processed food. It was I who was buying food loaded with sugar and grains. Max was addicted to corn chips and salsa after school and gluten free breakfast cereals. It was me buying gluten free bread for sandwiches, bagels, and gluten free chocolate chip cookies which in all reality are mostly carbs, sugar, corn, and potato starch. What was I thinking?

My son was not lacking antibiotics, steroids, and immune system suppressing drugs. My son was lacking real food, life supporting DHA found in wild fish such as sardines, mackerel, anchovies, herring, and sockeye salmon. CLA found in grass fed beef, bison, lamb, fresh raw milk, grass fed butter and cheese. My son was lacking probiotics found in homemade yogurt, good fats from avocados and coconut oil, essential minerals found in pistachios, almonds, walnuts, and lifesaving vitamins and antioxidants found in fresh organic fruits and vegetables.

However, Max was not able to digest any food at all. Trying to help my son who was losing weight daily and turning into a living skeleton, I called the hospital and asked the nurse to give us food recommendations for Max so that he can replace the nutrients, minerals, vitamins, proteins, and fats he had lost as a result of the diarrhea. Max was weak and malnourished but had the will to keep on going. His hair started to fall out because of lack of essential nutrients. They told me to come by and pick up a food sample the next day. They gave me a can of food manufactured in Ohio, by a company who makes infant formula for babies. So this was the best thing for my son? This liquid formula is very easy to digest and it contains all the essential amino-acids and nutrients that Max needs to get better. I was shocked. I was speechless. I could not believe it. The first ingredient on the list was high fructose corn syrup. How in the world could Max get any better by drinking corn syrup mixed with proteins derived from genetically modified soy beans and fats derived from corn and canola? I could not believe what was happening. What good was this can of food going to do for my son?

No wonder "two-thirds to three-quarters of patients with Crohn's disease will require surgery at some point during their lives. Surgery becomes necessary in Crohn's disease when medications can no longer control the symptoms" [36] - Centers for Disease Control and Prevention.

Control of the symptoms was not what Max was asking for. He was asking for a cure that would end his pain and suffering. How could I tell my twelve year old son that they did not have a cure for his medical condition and he has to live the rest of his life with this terrible disease. How could I tell my son that he is suffering because of me? Because of me being his miss-informed, health illiterate father without knowledge and wisdom, feeding his son grains and sugar instead of real food? Remember, knowledge and wisdom are everything.

I wish that the medical doctors knew more than me, but apparently they get their latest medical information watching TV commercials before bed time and promoting prescription drugs instead of real food. Do you think it is fun watching your son slowly bleed from ulcers inside his stomach and crippled from arthritis pain at only twelve?

OLD WORLD WISDOM

The next morning my old friend from Bosnia came to visit us. Seyfo is pushing his seventies. He is very strong built and is healthy for his age, standing six feet tall, sharp blue eyes, wide shoulders. He was trained as paratrooper back in the days and served as a translator for the US armed forces in Bosnia during the war in 1992-1995. Seyfo started crying when my twelve year old son entered the room. Max was skin and bones. His eyes had no spark. He was suffering from pain 24/7. The old man told me an amazing story that day about his mother, for she became very sick many years ago. "After being sick for a year, we lost hope in her recovery. We took her on a horse carriage in the middle of the winter to seek help from a famous physician practicing in another town. People were saying good things about this doctor". Seyfo was recalling events that happened over thirty years ago. "After six hours riding through the snow covered mountains in Bosnia we arrived at the university medical center. The doctor told my mother that he has one more recommendation for her, since they had no more prescription drugs to choose from. The doctor told us to buy a healthy goat and give my mother fresh raw goat milk every day for breakfast, for lunch and dinner. He told us to make yogurt, goat cheese and butter for her. Over the next seven months, my mother was healed. She fully recovered. Thanks to one physician in Bosnia who was not skeptical to prescribe food as a medicine against all the odds and all the criticism from the fellow medical doctors at the local university hospital".

I listened carefully to my friend's story and I could not find anything wrong with his testimony. After all, I remember from bible studies years ago, when the Israelites left Egypt with Moses they took all their sheep and all their goats with them. These animals were the only source for food for 2.5 million people wondering in the desert for forty years trying to find their way to the promised land, the land flowing with milk and honey, in Exodus 3:8. When the Israelites were to sacrifice the most precious possessions in their lives for forgiveness of sin, they would sacrifice their lamb and goats and bring them to the temple as their most precious offering to God who saved them from slavery and delivered them to the promised land.

I decided to do exactly what Seyfo told me, to find farm fresh raw goat milk and feed Max raw goat milk every day for breakfast, lunch, and dinner. The next morning I went to the Whole Foods Market to buy some raw goat milk. I was thinking if it is farm fresh I will be able to find there. When I arrived at the market I could not find any raw milk at all. They told me that they use to sell raw milk in the past but they cannot sell it anymore, because of the new regulations. Apparently selling raw milk is illegal business in California, I thought was a joke. I simply could not believe that all that fresh milk California produces has to be pasteurized or sterilized before sold. Unpasteurized milk is considered a health hazard in California. I was assured this was the only way to protect the public from milk contaminated with bacteria. This was so confusing to me, but I did find the truth behind this practice after doing some research. The truth is that many dairy farms today are practicing unsafe farming methods. The cows are raised indoors in a confined space, and fed cheap industrial processed animal feed, instead of healthy, organic hay. Many cows will eventually develop intestinal disease and diarrhea just like humans develop inflammatory bowel disease. The milk is frequently contaminated with bacteria found in cows feces and could be very dangerous to humans when consumed raw. But what about the small family farms that have a dozen of healthy goats and a dozen of healthy cows grazing on green pastures outdoors? Their milk is perfectly clean and needs no pasteurization. If the children on these small family farms can drink raw milk, why not share it with others in town, and sell the extra milk at the farmers market so we can buy some. The small family farm owners are not criminals. If their raw milk is good for their children on the farm, I want some for my children too.

Back in the nineties, Max's grandfather was the head of the dairy farms in Macedonia. The dairy farms and the milk processing industry were in big trouble so they appointed my father Mirko to make the necessary changes and improvements. He was an agriculture engineer with over 30 years of experience in the food processing industry. He said, "Saving the dairy industry was easy, but saving my grandson from industrial processed foods was extremely difficult".

Getting raw, farm fresh milk from Whole Foods was simply impossible. So I decided to find a good dairy farm where I could get the milk directly. Every farm I called and asked for raw milk denied my request. If you are a farmer in California you cannot sell raw milk and is illegal for me to buy raw milk. They told me the only way to get fresh raw goat milk in California is to buy or rent your own goat and drink your own milk. You will not break the law as long as you are not selling your milk to others. So, armed with new hope, I called another dozen dairy farmers in California asking to rent a goat so that I could get the milk for my son who is very sick and in desperate need of farm fresh goat milk. No dairy farm could accommodate my request claiming that they are booked at 100% and have no capacity nor they have government permit to take more co-op members. Renting a goat in California was impossible at the time so the only option left for me was to buy my own goat and bring to in the backyard of my house. I know it sounds crazy but I was desperate to find raw goat milk for my son.

A few days later, I finally received a phone call from a farm near San Diego, where I left a message for the owner a day before. The owner told me about a small family goat farm near San Francisco, that is licensed by the state of California to sell raw goat milk to the public.

Claravale Dairy Farm has been producing high quality raw goat milk for over 80 years. Thanks to the farm owner Dr. Ronald L. Garthwaite, BA, MA, PhD my son started drinking farm fresh raw goat milk from healthy goats in February of 2013. Six months later, without using any prescription drugs, Max completely recovered. We stopped all the prescription drugs the week after Max started drinking farm fresh raw goat milk. Max loved the fresh creamy taste of the cold milk. He was drinking a quart of the milk every day and gained back over 30 lbs. in the following six months. The goat milk and the home made yogurt was the only food that Max was able to digest in the beginning. In March of 2013, inspired by the book *Breaking The Vicious Cycle* [37] by Elaine Gottschall, we made the decision to change our family diet completely. We cleaned our kitchen of all the processed food, made with sugar and grain. No more processed food, milk, starches, grains, cereals, bread, pasta, donuts, cookies, and cakes. We removed all the food from our home that could potentially contain grain flour. All the snacks and all the packaged food in the house were gone in less than 30 minutes. There was not one single box of grain cereal left in the house. I will always remember that day. I saw the light at the end of the tunnel. We needed a fresh start so we bought a second refrigerator to stock pile on grass fed beef and lamb, wild Alaskan salmon, lamb chops, raw goat milk, homemade goat yogurt, homemade chicken bone stock, grass-fed butter, fresh fruits, fresh vegetables, pistachios, walnuts, almonds and hard cheeses aged to perfection. We started cooking with organic virgin coconut oil and cold pressed extra virgin olive oil for the salad dressings, mixed with organic apple cider vinegar, and Mediterranean sea salt. Not just for Max, but the entire family's diet and lifestyle had to change from high sugar diet to high fat diet rich in animal protein and essential fatty acids such as Omega-3 and CLA from pasture raised animals raised without any grains – grass fed, grass finished, beef and lamb.

On contrary of all doctors expectations that Max will live in pain for the rest of his life, Max completely recovered from Crohn's disease, without prescription drugs, in less than six months.

Blood sedimentation rate was reduced 20 times. From 61 mm/hr on 02/11/2013 to back to normal 3 mm/hr on 07/01/2013.

Fecal calprotectin protein (colon inflammation marker) was reduced 28 times. From 504 mcg/g on 12/20/2012 to back to normal 18 mch/g on 07/01/2013. The test was done at the Mayo Medical Laboratories testing site in North Carolina, less than six months after Max diet was changed from processed foods made with grains and sugar, to farm-fresh real food. This farm-fresh real food is high in dietary cholesterol, high in CLA, high in Omega-3 essential fatty acids from wild fish and pasture raised animals - grass fed grass finished beef and lamb.

"Let food be thy medicine and medicine be thy food"- Hippocrates.

Blood C-reactive protein (inflammation marker) was reduced 12 times. From 6.2 mg/dl on 02/11/2013 to back to normal 0.5 mg/dl on 07/01/2013 in less than six months after changing his diet to farm fresh real food - no grains, no sugar, no starches.

We were told so many times "There is no medical cure for Crohn's disease" and they were absolutely right because the cure is at the farm and not at the pharmacy. Crohn's disease and many other inflammatory, degenerative autoimmune diseases are without medical cure. Fortunately they are life style driven and can be avoided and sometimes even reversed by completely changing your diet and lifestyle. I don't know if Max is cured in medical terms, but he is definitely inflammation and pain free and always will be as long as he stays on his diet plan - **grain free and sugar free real food.**

The food that our ancestors ate for thousands of years is good for you. It is real food. The beef they ate was pasture raised not corn fed. The fish they ate was wild caught not farm raised. The food our ancestors ate was beyond organic, clean, never processed, never altered, real food. Today we live in a different world surrounded by processed food and genetically modified food. We had no other choice but to eliminate all food made with grains and sugar.

Inspired by solid medical evidence published in the most prestigious peer reviewed medical journals in the past 24 months, we managed to reset the clock one hundred years back to 1913 when chronic inflammatory diseases such as Crohn's did not exist, when processed foods were not invented yet, when corn was not genetically modified and raw goat milk was legal in California.

GLYCATION OF PROTEINS

I can have donuts, caramel macchiato, cupcakes, pizza, granola-bars, honey-nut breakfast cereals, milkshakes, ice-cream and never get sick. This was my point of view before 2013. Many scientific research papers were published in the past five years and new diagnostic tools were developed, revealing the real causes for inflammation in the human body. Highly processed foods and excess sugar consumption are deadly combination. For most physicians this means business as usual. Physicians have no time to read medical research papers and even if they do have time to read, there is no medicine your doctor can prescribe to change your lifestyle or to lower your daily sugar intake. What you eat is your choice. It is up to you.

You don't have to be a medical doctor to read the statistics. Today one out of four people in the U.S. dies prematurely with a coronary heart disease. The first symptom for coronary heart disease is usually a heart attack and a sudden death. The autopsy follows right after the first symptom and it reveals inflammation and blocked coronary arteries. Crohn's disease on the other side starts as inflammation in the digestive organs and the pain and suffering can last for decades. Both medical conditions are without medical cure, because they are life style driven. My son developed inflammatory degenerative disease because I was buying processed food instead of real food. The American Heart Association recommends not more than 100 calories a day from sugar if you are a woman and not more than 150 calories a day from sugar if you are a man.[2] Why did I chose grain and sugar loaded food for my son? Because the food was cheap and addictive, because I was not informed how dangerous it is, and because I had no knowledge about real food such as wild fish and pasture raised beef raised without grains, without hormones, without antibiotics, without <u>cattle feed additives</u>, and without <u>zilpaterol.</u> Our children need real food to function properly, physically, psychologically, and socially. I had to learn fast, to help my son. It is not that complicated. If you want to get sick, this is the formula that is proven to work for my family:

grains + sugar + Omega 6 = chronic inflammation and pain

According to <u>OECD</u> we as Americans are currently spending $7,960.00 per person, per year for health care, totaling about $2.5 trillion dollars per year, the U.S. government currently contributing 46% of the money or $1.13 trillion dollars per year in tax payer money for hospital beds and prescription drugs. This kind of health care spending [38] is going to bankrupt our economy as we are eating more processed foods than ever, getting sicker in return. "Between 1970 and 2010, health care spending quintupled as a percent of our federal budget. As a percent of GDP, health care spending is now projected to double in the next 25 years", "For the first time in the US history this generation of children is expected to have shorter life expectancy then their parents" [1] These statistics are unacceptable for the most prosperous nation in the world. I believe that the truth will save our nation or at least this generation. Here is the formula that is proven to work for my family:

no grains + no sugar + Omega 3 + CLA = no inflammation, no pain

The excess grain and sugar consumption is spreading worldwide causing obesity and inflammatory chronic conditions not just in the elderly but also in young children like Max. The blood glucose binds with different proteins in the body in a process called "protein glycation". Oxidants can further chemically modify these "glycated proteins" producing advanced glycation end-products or AGEs. [18] The accumulation of these modified proteins can be a factor in the development or worsening of many chronic inflammatory conditions. These harmful compounds called advanced glycation end-products can affect nearly every cell and molecule in the body. The symptoms are inflammation, chronic pain, and degeneration of organs in the body. Listen to your body. If you already have aches and pains your body is telling you something very important: you are aging fast and the cells in your body do not have time to repair and regenerate. You need real food instead of sugar and grains. Protein glycation, premature aging, and chronic inflammation are directly related to sugar consumption.

The truth about protein glycation was published in 2013 in Germany by Andreas Simm with the Department of Cardiothoracic Surgery at University Hospital in Halle, Germany. [39]

The research paper Protein glycation during aging and in cardiovascular disease [39] was published in a Special Issue of Journal of Proteomics, Volume 92, October 30, 2013, Pages 248-259. A few months later, Andreas Simm published another research paper together with a group of German scientists, about the role of advanced glycation end-products in cellular signaling · The paper was published in Redox Biology, Volume 2, January 9, 2014, Pages: 411-429. This research paper is available at the US National Library of Medicine. [40]

The new medical studies confirm glucose - blood sugar being directly linked to glycation of proteins, inflammation and aging in your body. In my personal opinion, Crohn's disease was nothing else but the most extreme manifestation of malnutrition, inflammation and premature aging.

Find a physician trained in functional medicine and check your blood C-reactive protein inflammation markers regularly. Eliminate all processed foods, sugar and grains from your diet. Enjoy raw fruits, nuts, and green vegetables (sautéed in garlic butter for example) instead of grains.

Real food is the best choice not only for the sick, but also for healthy, professional athletes who need to be in top shape 24/7. Reducing inflammation means no more pain in your joints after the game. It means clear vision and a clear mind, a happy mood and lots of energy all day long. No sugar crash ever again. For breaking new records you need to break the old sweet habits.

Instead of sugar, your body and brain will be running on Omega-3 found in real food, grass-fed butter, cheese, homemade yogurt, wild fish, walnuts, virgin coconut oil, pasture raised poultry [77], farm fresh eggs [80], grass-fed beef [81], and pasture raised lamb[82]

Recommended reading Molecular Metabolism Volume 3, Issue 2, [83] Pages 94-108
http://www.sciencedirect.com/science/article/pii/S2212877813001245

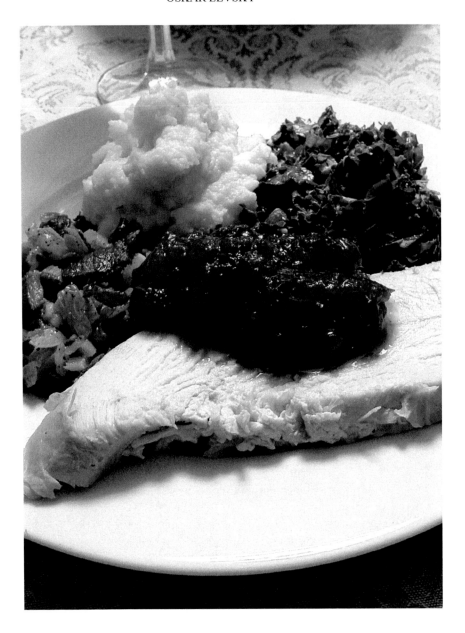

Grain and sugar free dinner plate. Ingredients: cauliflower puree, kale, pasture raised turkey, sautéed onions, walnuts, resins, sugar free bacon, celery, organic carrots, olive oil, coconut oil, garlic, sea salt, black pepper, cranberries, butter, honey, grapefruit juice, and lemon juice.

In 1765 a man by the name of Boulanger, opened a shop near the Louvre in Paris, France. There he sold what he called "bouillons restaurants", that is meat based consommés intended to "restore" a person's strength. [41]

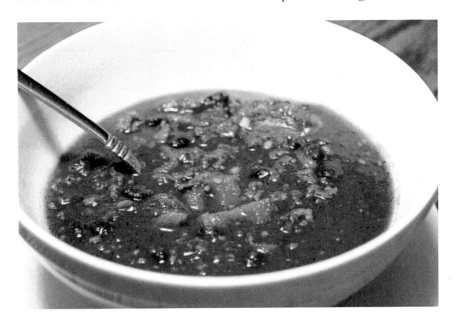

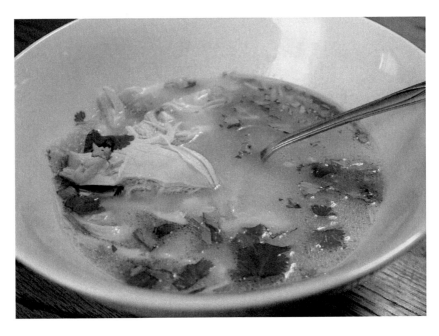

RAW GOAT MILK

Raw milk has different properties then pasteurized milk. Once heated, milk becomes rotten with precipitated minerals that cannot be absorbed (hence osteoporosis), with sugars that cannot be digested (hence allergies), and with fats that are toxic. Raw milk from grass fed healthy animals has been used as a therapy in folk medicine (and even at the Mayo Clinic) for centuries. It has been used in the pre-insulin days to treat diabetes (I've tried it - it works) as well as eczema, intestinal worms, allergies, and arthritis, all for reasons which can be understood when we realize just what is in the raw milk - Thomas Cowan, MD. [42]

Goat milk in its raw form is nature's perfect food. It has a complete protein complex that contains all the essential amino acids. If you have ever been on a farm, you would notice that goats are much more flexible and happier than cows. They climb everywhere and do things that are beautiful and fun to watch. You have seen goats get on the roofs of barns and farm houses and you wondered how was that possible. The reason for this is that goats are special and very different then cows. [43]

Bio-organic sodium is known in Naturopathic Medicine as the youth element and the deficiency of this essential mineral is associated with arthritis. Many adults but also children today suffer with inflammatory, degenerative and autoimmune disease. What you did not know is that the best sources of bio-organic sodium is found in raw goat milk. It is the bio-organic sodium that keeps the goats young, active, flexible, and limber all of their lives. They will always climb, jump, leap, and even climb trees because the bio-organic sodium is the mobilizing material that makes this possible. [43]

Each organ of the body has a reserve of one chemical element more than other organs. This principle, known as "the chemical story" is one of the essential principles of the Naturopathic Medicine. The stomach is known as a bio-organic sodium organ in naturopathic medicine. When the body becomes deficient in bio-organic sodium, foods do not digest properly. The stomach's ability to produce enzymes and hydrochloric acid is slowed down and we experience belching, bloating, and ulcers with many other digestive problems. Coffee, tea, sugar, white flour products, chocolate, alcohol, and especially soda drinking produces high stomach acid imbalance that absorbs the bioorganic sodium right off the walls of the stomach and colon. This condition sometimes takes many years to manifest itself and is not noticed until it becomes a named disease. **Raw milk was used successfully as a medical therapy in America** before the war by Dr. J.R. Crewe, MD [44]

Disclaimer: These statements have not been evaluated by the US Food and Drug Administration (FDA). To prevent our food from being classified as drugs under Section 201(g) of the Federal Food, Drug and Cosmetic Act, we are required to inform you that there is no intention, implied or otherwise that represents or infers that these food products or statements be used in the cure, diagnosis, mitigation, treatment, or prevention of any disease.

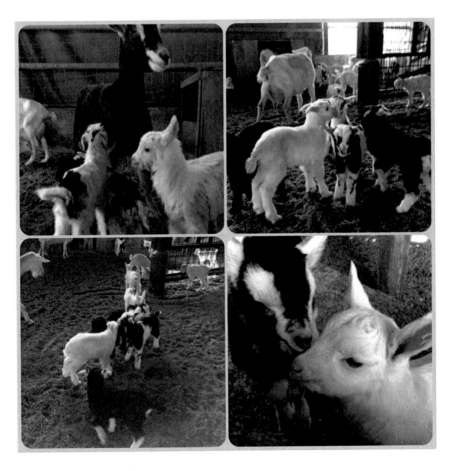

http://www.yagimilk.com/

"The milk consumed in biblical times differed much from the milk we consume today. The milk of the Bible came from cows and goats and was consumed straight from the animal or it was immediately fermented. Goat's milk alkalizes the digestive system. It actually contains an alkaline ash, and it does not produce acid in the intestinal system. Goat's milk helps to increase the pH of the blood stream because it is the dairy product highest in the amino acid L-glutamine." -excerpt from the book *The Maker's Diet* pages *147-149,* by Jordan Rubin.[45]

Jordan Rubin's Beyond Organic Farm in Southern Missouri [46] goes far and beyond the organic standards for farming and growing organic food. "Our animals are GreenFed™ and GreenFinished™" - Jordan Rubin. "Our dairy cattle intensely graze on grasses and a "salad bar" of forbs, herbs, and legumes – with no grains. Our beef cattle partake in our green finishing program, which includes a bovine detoxification program and a diet of fresh organic pasture supplemented in the winter with green foods such as alfalfa and certified organic hay with no grain." [47]

The Owner of Claravale Dairy, Dr. Ron Garthwaite, BA, MA, PhD has helped thousands of children like my son rebuilding their nutrient depleted bodies with essential and easy to digest nutrients, probiotics and enzymes found only in not processed raw goat milk. [49.] http://claravaledairy.com/ The California state government instead of recognizing these highly responsible farmers for their extraordinary work and contribution to society, they have decided to pressure them and put the farmers out of business by making false claims that their raw milk is not safe. As I've explained already, the problem with raw milk is not the milk, but the people who take care of the animals. Pasteurization cannot protect you from irresponsible farmers. Choose your dairy farm wisely. Check the farm history with the local USDA office, the local chamber of commerce and the better business bureau. Make sure they are running a clean farming operation.[48] http://www.organicpastures.com/

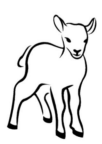

Raw goat milk is the best choice for nourishing a sick person back to health. That is why we need to have access to farm fresh raw milk just like we need to have access to farm fresh raw fruits, vegetables, eggs, meats. However, drinking contaminated raw milk is very dangerous. That is why we choose to drink clean milk from inspected, healthy, disease-free goats that are raised with love and care [51]

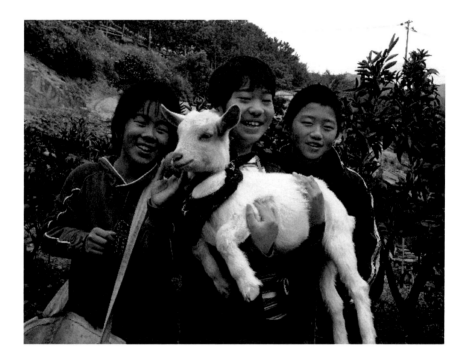

http://www.yagimilk.com/

HOME MADE YOGURT

So what do you do if you can't find raw milk since most states including California have outlawed the sale of raw milk for human consumption, even with research showing all its amazing benefits? The entire yogurt we have made at home for Max was made with farm fresh raw goat milk from Claravale Dairy Farm. So what do you do if you cannot find fresh raw goat milk in your state? Well, you need to move out from that state or you need to reverse the law in the state you live in. For many U.S. citizens, homemade yogurt from pasteurized milk is the only option they have besides moving out of the state. Homemade yogurt offers similar benefits to raw milk. However, regardless of how many television commercials you have seen in the past featuring the benefits of commercially made yogurt please take my advice today and just forget about television and start making your own yogurt.

The Greeks make their yogurt at home using two ingredients: 1. fresh milk 2. live yogurt culture. They enjoy long healthy life for a reason. Everywhere you go in Greece and especially on the beautiful Greek islands, you will see many old but healthy people, eating and drinking all day long with their friends and family. Their diet is mostly catch of the day, grass fed lamb, goat milk, goat yogurt, feta cheese (sheep milk), vine ripened tomatoes, pickled olives, farm fresh eggs, olive oil, cucumbers and nothing more. The Greeks do not eat fast food nor junk food like the rest of Europe. You can enjoy the benefits of a homemade yogurt too. It is actually very easy to make. You can turn the milk into live food by adding the original pro-biotic yogurt culture (L.bulgaricus, S.thermopilus, L.acidophilus) to make yogurt at home. Make sure the milk is from grass-fed animals whenever possible. This is important because the concentration of CLA in the milk is five times higher when you drink grass-fed milk and yogurt.

Being raised on green pastures is critical for the health of the animal and for the quality of the milk. Sheep, goats and cows were created to graze on green pastures. Grass-fed dairy cows and goats produce milk that has amazing taste. Once you have had a glass of fresh raw milk from Claravale Dairy Farm in California, you will never go back to commodity milk. However, less than 3% of all cattle in the U.S. are grass-fed and there are only two USDA accredited farms in California that have a state license to produce and sell raw milk.

I love my grandmother Fotia. She is 84 and still making her yogurt at home every week. She has 7 children, 13 grandchildren and 15 great grandchildren. If it is Greek, it should only have two ingredients according to my grandma Fotia (Φωτια = Fire) born in Thessaloniki, Greece in 1929. The Greek yogurt is not a desert my grandmother explains. The yogurt is not supposed to have any sugar nor thickening agents added in it. We use to make it every day, from fresh (raw) milk, for thousands of years in Greece. The purpose of drinking yogurt is to keep you hydrated and nourished with all the essential nutrients and electrolytes that you need during the hot days while working in the vineyards or fishing at open sea. It keeps your body alkaline; it keeps you hydrated all day long. The yogurt is served cold with every meal, for breakfast, for lunch and at the dinner table as a "tzatziki sauce" served with grilled meats. It is made of strained yogurt from sheep or goat milk, mixed with cucumbers, garlic, salt and olive oil.

HOME MADE YOGURT, INGREDIENTS:

1. farm fresh whole milk (preferable raw milk from a healthy goat, sheep or cow)
2. active live yogurt culture (L.bulgaricus, S.thermopilus, L.acidophilus)

COMMERCIALLY MADE YOGURT:

1. Cultured Pasteurized Nonfat Milk
2. Milk Protein Concentrate,
3. Sugar,
4. Pectin
5. Gelatin
6. Lemon Juice Concentrate,
7. Natural Flavor,
8. Locust Bean Gum,
9. Vitamin A Acetate,
10. Vitamin D3

When I was growing up, I remember my grandmother making yogurt for us. The success was measured by how thick and creamy the yogurt was. Not always the yogurt would came out perfect, but it is very simple to make one at home, using controlled temperature 42-44°C (108-112°F) and timing 6-24 hrs. When you are sick you need real food. You cannot have sugar and food additives and expect to get better. Everything you eat must be pure and natural, not modified, not changed, and not altered.

Everything you purchase needs to be farm fresh, not modified, just like your ancestors eat for thousands of years and maintained their healthy alkaline body structure without arthritis, cancer, heart disease. The most important part of your recovery is to keep your body alkaline, hydrated and nourished. Give your immune system a chance to repair itself, that means eliminate sugar, starches and grains from your diet completely. The homemade yogurt contains billions of beneficial microorganisms called probiotics [84.]

Scientists have identified over 500 different strains of beneficial bacteria that coexist in your body. [54] Every one of these friendly bacteria has a different purpose to complete a specific task and keep you healthy and nourished. Every person has a different combination of these peace keeping solders living inside of your gut. Dr. Jeffry Gordon's research [52] shows that we have ten times more bacteria in us then the total amount of human cells we are made of. With other words we are mostly made of bacteria and only 10% human cells.[53] "Microbes Keep Us Alive" explains Dr. Jeffrey Gordon director of the Center for Genome Sciences at Washington University - St. Louis School of Medicine. [52, 53, 54]

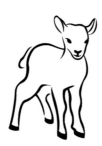

PASTURE RAISED BEEF AND LAMB

My father Mirko was the head of the dairy industry in Macedonia from 1985 to 1992. That means all the major dairy farms in the country were managed by his office. Being an agricultural engineer since 1966 he had more experience in food production and food processing than I will ever have. He knows all about commercial dairy farms operations and turning milk into yogurt, cheese, cream, butter, etc. He knows all about turning beef into cash which is apparently impossible, unless you feed the cattle cheap animal feed and additives such as zilpaterol and ractopamine to promote growth of muscle mass.

I asked him to help me understand why the beef has a bad reputation, and is being associated with high blood pressure and high cholesterol? Apparently, less than 5% of the beef in the USA is "grass fed - grass finished". This means less than 5% of the beef cattle is raised outdoors, grazing on green pastures, enjoying forbs, herbs and legumes. Today over 95% of the beef comes from commercial beef feedlots where the beef cattle is fed special combination of greens, grains and feed additives.

Lactic Acidosis, known as grain poisoning in farm animals is common feedlot nutritional disorder which can affect animals that consume too much starch or sugar in a short period of time. [55] Their lipid profile is totally different compared to pasture raised, grass-fed grass-finished beef, grandpa explained. These animals usually spend their last three to six months in feedlots, during which time they gain between two and four pounds per day by eating lots of grains, including genetically modified grains containing the chemical glyphosate responsible for cancer in laboratory animals. [56] Beside eating lots of grains these animals are fed special feed additives to promote muscle growth such as <u>zilpaterol</u> [57] and <u>ractopamine</u>. [58] Few days before slaughter, they have to stop using these beta agonist drugs to protect beef consumers around the world being exposed to. On December 7, 2012 Russia's Federal Agency for Agricultural Control, banned the imports of all meat containing ractopamine. This is a cattle feed additive that allows to reduce the content of fat in beef. The drug is added to the animal feed so that animals grow more muscle mass instead of fat. <u>The drug is banned for use in 160 countries</u>. It is is allowed in 24 countries including Canada and the United States. [59]

According to grandpa, Max needed real food - pasture raised beef, lamb, mutton, and wild fish such as wild Alaskan salmon, sardines, mackerels, anchovies, herrings. Max needs lots of Omega-3 fatty acids, that are essential for reducing inflammation in his body, grandpa explained.

Pasture raised beef has 30% less calories and 400% more <u>CLA</u> compared to grain-fed beef coming from beef feedlots. The ratio of Omega-6 over Omega-3 in grass fed beef is 2:1 compared to grain fed beef being 18:1 Being rich in Omega-3 and CLA, pasture raised beef and lamb helps with inflammation in the body.

CLA on the other side is <u>cancer fighting</u> poly-unsaturated fatty acid found in highest concentrations in pasture raised grass fed grass finished beef and lamb. <u>CLA</u> has been shown to modulate immune functions in diabetic and cancer patients. It was discovered in 1987 by Michael Pariza. Animal studies shows that as little as 0.5 percent CLA in your diet could reduce tumors by over 50 percent, including breast, colorectal, lung, skin, and stomach cancer. [60]

Over the past 26 years over 400 medical research papers were published on the health benefits of CLA - Conjugated Linoleic Acid. [61] Many research papers are available online for free at the <u>US National Library of Medicine</u>.

"Let food be thy medicine and medicine be thy food"- Hippocrates 460-370 B.C. [62]

"Cows grazing pasture and receiving no supplemental feed had <u>500% more conjugated linoleic acid</u> in milk fat than cows fed typical dairy diets". [63]

Pasture raised, grass fed, grass finished beef

<u>www.uswellnessmeats.com</u>

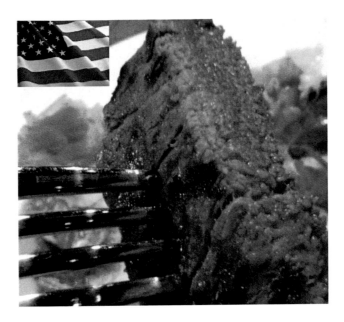

New Zealand's sheep and cattle are raised in free-range open fields year-round, and live on a natural diet of fresh pasture, grass and nutrient-rich clover - eliminating the need for grain feeding and nutritional supplements. A focus on healthy animals living in good conditions is at the heart of the New Zealand meat industry. Pasture-fed and naturally raised meat has a unique, internationally sought-after flavor. New Zealand has a sophisticated meat industry that produces outstanding, pasture-fed and naturally raised meat. The products are tender, flavorful, healthy and customized for clients around the world. New Zealand has an almost exclusively free-range grass feed production system producing tender, appetizing and healthy products.[64]

No grain-feeding, No feed-additives

New Zealand livestock's diet of fresh pasture, grass and nutrient-rich clover almost completely eliminates grain-feeding and nutritional supplementation.

And, with strict bio-security and quality control processes, our animals produce not only tasty but extremely healthy and safe meat. [64]

The New Zealand red meat sector has been a principal driver of New Zealand's economy and identity, generating nearly NZ $8 billion annually in export earnings. The industry enjoys a unique combination of competitive advantages - industry knowledge gained from a long history as farmers, world-leading research and development and support infrastructure, and stringent bio-security standards. The combination of these factors allows New Zealand to stand ahead of its competitors and consistently improve its reputation for quality and innovation in the global market.

Organic sheep and beef

New Zealand red meat exporters are integrating their marketing with overseas retailers to provide out-of-season product for the northern hemisphere. New Zealand has growing organic sheep and beef industries, operating under standards developed by private sector accreditation organizations such as Bio-Gro. [64]

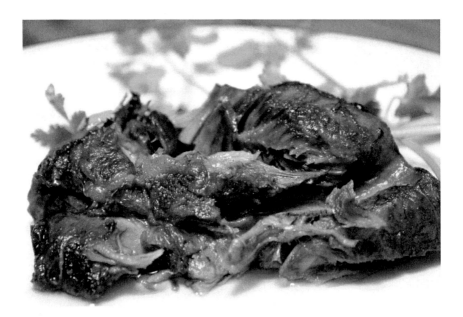

NEW ZEALAND LAMB

Disease-Free Animals

New Zealand maintains its reputation as a safe and secure supply source. Any major incursions are quickly contained and controlled, minimizing longer-term negative impacts on New Zealand exports. New Zealand's strict bio-security controls and geographic isolation have resulted in an animal disease-free status, recognized by the World Organization for Animal Health. [64]

Traceable Livestock

Electronic databases have been used by New Zealand farmers for over 10 years, enabling each animal to be recorded from conception to export. This system is being expanded with the National Animal Identification and Traceability Project (NAIT) implemented in 2012. NAIT is a robust electronic system, which individually tags livestock with electronic ear tags. [64] In the event of a bio-security alert, infected animals can be quickly identified and traced by their individual tag number, location and the person responsible for that animal. The scheme is mandatory for cattle from 1 July 2012, and for deer from 1 March 2013.

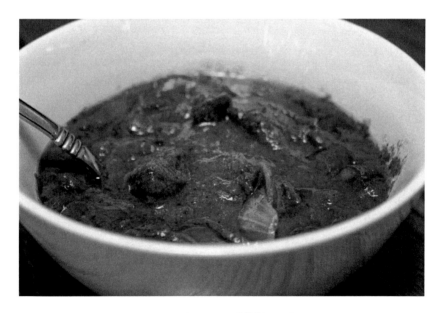

SPICY MASALA MUTTON CURRY

Food Safety Standards

New Zealand sets the highest standards for its food producers to ensure that the country remains a world leader in food safety. The New Zealand Food Safety Authority (NZFSA) is responsible for New Zealand's food-related legislation. Around 200,000 export certificates are issued annually by the NZFSA for animal products. [64]

Animal health and breeding

New Zealand's sheep and cattle are raised in free-range open fields year-round, and live on a natural diet of fresh pasture, grass and nutrient-rich clover - eliminating the need for grain feeding and nutritional supplements. A temperate climate also means animals do not need energy-intensive housing during the winter months. Animal welfare standards in New Zealand are exceptionally high and are protected by legislation. [64]

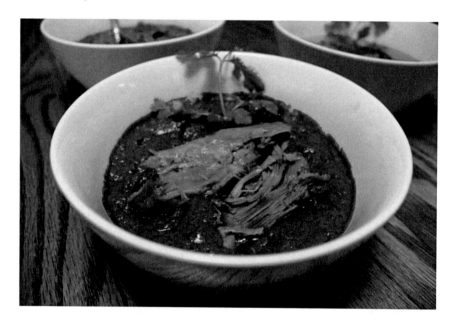

ORGANIC SPINACH CURRY

JAPAN'S NATIONAL LIVING TREASURE

Nobody takes their food and health more seriously than the people of Japan. The Japanese spend three times more income on food, then on housing. The Americans on contrary, spend three times more income on housing then on food.

Japan's small family farms are beautiful, clean, organized and very competitive. You can order garden fresh Japanese apples and sweet melons through the post office website and have it delivered to you together with your regular mail. The post office in Japan actually makes profit selling real food instead of post-stamps. The small family farms in Japan grow the world best quality fruits and vegetables. The dark volcanic soil is rich in nutrients and the quality of the produce is simply amazing. The goal of every family farm in Japan is to produce the best quality regardless of the cost and regardless of the market price. Producing cheap food was never the plan for the Japanese farmers.

The world best tasting beef comes also from Japan. Kobe Beef refers to cuts of beef from the Tajima strain of Wagyu cattle, raised in Hyogo Prefecture, according to rules set by the Kobe Beef Marketing & Distribution Promotion Association. [65] Kyoto is the capital of the Hyogo Prefecture and my favorite city in Japan. Waguy is considered to be delicacy, renowned for its flavor, tenderness, superior fat content and well-marbled texture. [66] Realizing the value of their unique local product the government ceased all exports of Wagyu cattle and declared them a national living treasure protected by law in Japan. A 14-ounce Wagyu Rib Eye Steak from Japan sell for $310 in a steak house in Hong Kong. [66]

However, these days for the first time in Japan's history, the Japanese young people are moving away from the traditional Japanese cuisine. Instead of enjoying their unique quality food, grown locally on a small family farms, this generation of young people wants cheap processed foods made with gluten, grains and sugar. Every time I go shopping for food in Tokyo, I look at the shopping carts of the Japanese people going up and down the escalator. Saving money on food is always a bad choice. Buying processed food made with sugar and grains instead of beef, lamb, mutton, salmon, and mackerel will have tremendous negative impact on the health of this generation, unless they change their lifestyle and turn back to traditional Japanese food as described in this chapter. For thousands of years, the local small family farms in Japan have been supplying high quality food, wild fish, beef, fresh milk, grass-fed butter, pasture raised chicken, eggs, and variety of fresh fruits and vegetables. The quality and the freshness of the locally grown food in Japan is out of this world and it is not cheap. I have never had better tasting apples, strawberries, tomatoes and carrots in my life. There is no national cuisine that can come even close when it comes to food quality and food taste. When it comes to your health knowledge about real food is everything.

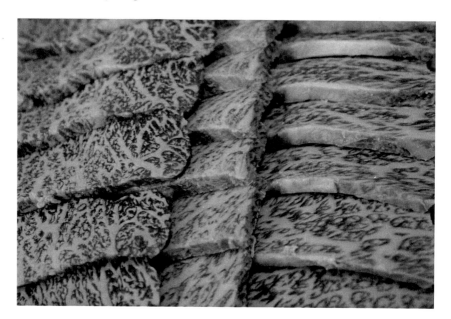

JAPAN NATIONAL INSTITUTE
OF HEALTH AND NUTRITION

March 11, 2014 "A diet high in protein, particularly animal protein, may help elderly individuals function at higher levels physically, psychologically, and socially", according to a new study by <u>Megumi Tsubota-Utsugi, PhD</u> and her colleagues in Tohoku University and Teikyo University. [68]

JAPANESE CUISINE WINS
CULTURAL HERITATE STATUS

December 5, 2013 "Washoku" traditional Japanese cuisine has been added to UNESCO's Intangible Cultural Heritage list, raising the government's hopes of enhancing its global recognition, attracting more foreign tourists and boosting exports of the country's agricultural products. "We are truly happy," Prime Minister Shinzo Abe said of the UNESCO recognition in a statement released Thursday morning. "We would like to continue passing on Japanese food culture to the generations to come". [67]

Locally grown, farm fresh food is the key for the health of the nation. The nation's economy is strong only when the people are healthy. People are healthy only when they have access to farm-fresh organic fruits and vegetables, grass fed beef and lamb, pasture raised chicken, eggs, fresh raw milk, yogurt, butter, cheese. The key is to keep your body alkaline, toxin free and inflammation free. Locally grown farm fresh food, cooked at home instead of factory processed food means very few hospital visits in your lifetime.

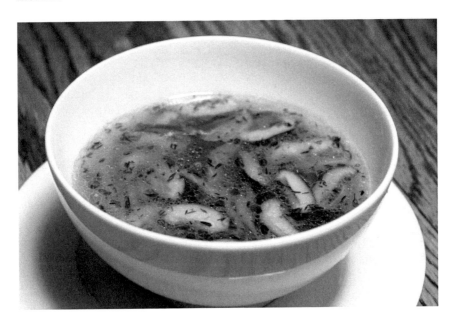

GRAIN FREE SHITAKE MUSHROOM SOUP

AFFORDABLE HEALTH CARE

The Children Hospital Los Angeles diagnosed my son with Crohn's Disease. The cost of diagnostics and doctor's visits was about $10,000. The Claravale Dairy Farm supplied us with farm fresh raw goat milk. The cost of the fresh raw goat milk was $64 a week or $1664 over six months during Max's recovery. We also spent additional $8,000 on grass-fed beef, pasture raised chicken, farm-fresh eggs, cheese, raw-nuts, locally grown organic fruits and vegetables. Yes, we spent about $9,664.00 on farm fresh organic food over six months, but we also saved about $398,000 by avoiding grains, sugar, proscription drugs, hospitalizations, and surgeries.

Chronic inflammatory diseases such as diabetes, high blood pressure, heart disease, and joint deterioration, what were once considered adult diseases, are regularly being diagnosed in children today. These are life style driven health conditions and can be avoided. They cost our economy $2.5 trillion dollars each year - watch video [69]. The solution to this problem is bringing back to life the small family farms that are going to supply farm fresh real food instead of hospital beds. The small family farms and their grass-fed livestock, should be the fastest growing segment of our economy and they should be protected by law as a national treasure.

- Some of the medical research data shows that people with high cholesterol live the longest according to Dr. Harlan Krumholz, MD with the department of Cardiovascular Medicine at Yale University. [6]

- Stephanie Seneff, PhD, talks about cholesterol sulfate deficiency in her latest research paper published in 2013 in Entropy, Volume 15, Issue 4, Pages 1416-1463. [7]

- Dr. David Perlmutter, MD talks about cholesterol benefits in his new book published in 2013, Grain Brain - The surprising truth about wheat, carbs and sugar - your brain's silent killers. [8]

- Thomas Gawlowski explains advanced glycation and cardio vascular effects. Understanding the pathogenic mechanisms of AGEs is paramount to develop strategies against diabetic and cardiovascular complications. [83]

SMALL PELAGIC OPEN OCEAN FISH

There are hundreds of scientific papers published in the past 50 years on the health benefits of fish oil - DHA essential fatty acids find in fish. Finally everybody, the medical doctors, the insurance companies, the hospitals, the patients, and even the pharmaceutical companies agree that the nutrition properties of fish oil are essential for human health and immune system support. The Omega-3 fatty acids are anti-inflammatory, meaning more fish you have in your diet, less chances you have to develop inflammatory heart disease, inflammatory bowel disease, and inflammatory arthritis, less chances for dementia and memory loss.[70]

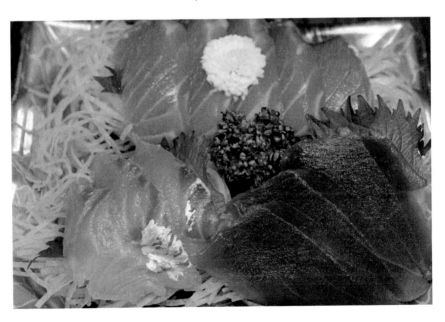

However be aware, because not all fish is good for you and some are banned for human consumption.[70] The fish that our ancestors ate and the fish we farm today are not the same. The new farming practices and the water pollution will have direct impact on the fish you eat and on your health. When it comes to salmon, always look for wild Alaskan salmon or

Sockeye salmon. When it comes to tuna fish be aware that the contamination with mercury in big fish, such as tuna and marlin, could be thousand times higher compared to the small but clean and healthy sardine's mackerels, anchovies, herrings. DHA is the most effective natural therapy when it comes to inflammation in your body. DHA is an omega-3 fatty acid that is the primary structural component of the human brain. You should be getting minimum 1,000 mg of DHA every day by consuming wild fish, sardines, mackerels, anchovies, herrings, wild salmon and pasture raised beef.

A recent study published on July 1st, 2013 found that DHA is used to produce maresins in the body which fights inflammation. "We've known for a long time that DHA tames inflammation, now, we learn exactly how DHA works: via new substances called maresins," - said Gerald Weissmann, M.D.[72]

Sardines, Mackerels, Anchovies, Herrings, are clean fish and excellent source of Omega-3 and very popular around the world, but especially in Japan. They belong to a category called small pelagic open ocean fish; they live near the surface but never on the bottom of the sea. They are biblical clean fish with scales and fins, not scavengers, not bottom feeders. Stay away from bottom feeders - their job is to clean the ocean floor from dead animals, and digest whatever they can find on the bottom of the ocean as if they were vacuum cleaners.

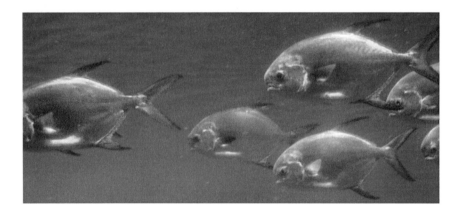

BONE MARROW STOCK

My grandmother Rebekah would come back home every night with a bag of beef bones for our dog Jackie. I was only five years old and had no clue where these bones came from. Sixteen years ago when my daughter Rebekah was born, grandma explained to me about the bones. Grandma was working as a chef at The Children's Hospital in Skopje - Macedonia. She would leave her home before sunrise and Jackie, our black Labrador, would walk with her to the hospital to make her company even when the ground was covered with three foot of snow. Grandma would start cooking for the children as early as 4:30 AM every morning. She would boil beef bones for 24 hours and make a nutritious beef stock. The next day she would use the beef stock in every meal she created for the children at the hospital. There was no such food as corn-flex or oat cereal in Macedonia, except for the horses. Day in and day out, after two-three months on grandma's high fat, high cholesterol, Omega-3 diet (grain and sugar free) the children would leave the hospital healthy. Most of the children at the hospital had Tuberculosis and had to be hospitalized for weeks and months. Our black Labrador Jackie was the luckiest dog in town, enjoying beef bone marrow and cartilage from grass-fed beef bones every day of his dog life.

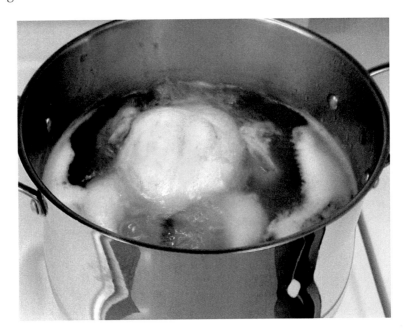

These days in America nobody has the time for cooking good food for the children, never the less for the dogs. But in reality, you can turn on the crock pot in the morning before you go to work and enjoy fantastic pasture raised chicken or lamb tonight. I make my chicken stock over the weekend. For chicken stock, you need to boil the bones for 12 hours to make good inflammation fighting chicken stock. All the good nutrients from the bones, including **bone marrow, cartilage, gelatin, glucosamine, collagen**, will be extracted over 12 hours of slow simmering in your kitchen. There is no pharmacy in the world that can do this process better then you. It is not that complicated and you do not need a degree in chemistry.

After getting the stock to boiling, you can turn the heat down and check every 6 hours. Just make sure you have really big stainless steel (not aluminum) pot and enough water in it to cover the bones. If you want to have a healthy family this is the only way to get the nutrients your body needs to function and perform. Once it cools down, the broth will turn into gelatin. That is a good sign that you have learned the art of making stock. The art of making bone stock is one of the most valuable properties of French and Japanese traditional cooking. Now you can use the chicken stock in every meal you'll create during the week for you and your family.

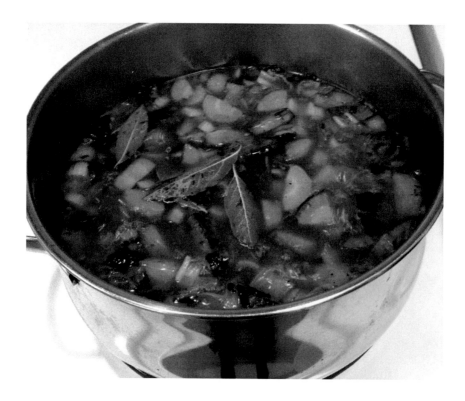

To have young , performing, healthy body, you will need good nutrition. From Paris to Tokyo every good meal starts with homemade bone stock. There is nothing better for your good health and flexible joints as you are growing older. Learn how to make beef stock, chicken stock, fish stock. It will change your life by reducing inflammation in your body.

In August 2013 Max had his last health check at the Children's Hospital LA He was completely symptoms free. Grandma Marika flew from Macedonia to help us in the kitchen. She was in charge for breakfast, lunch and dinner seven days a week for six months, making sure Max is getting all the nutrition he needs. Against all odds and expectations Max's Crohn's disease was completely reversed in less than six months on real food. [75]

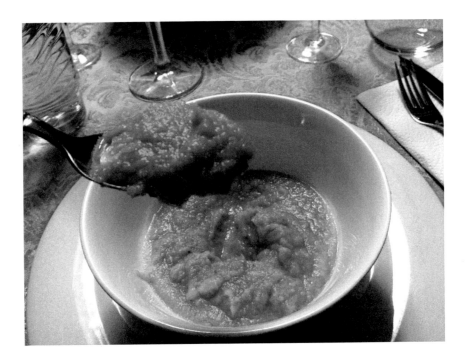

When you are diagnosed with chronic inflammatory disease, when you are in pain and your inflammation is 28 times beyond the normal levels, you are going to need professional medical help. You need to talk to your doctor. Together you need to choose the right food and the right medicine, because when the inflammation sets in your body, the pain and the suffering are unbearable.

Most medical doctors born in the city, never had a homemade chicken soup, cooked the old fashioned way, simmering in the kitchen for many hours on low heat, using pasture raised whole chicken, and adding garden fresh vegetables, carrots, celery, parsley, sage, rosemary, thyme, cilantro, see salt, black pepper.

All you are going to need is more room in your refrigerator for farm fresh food, regardless of which part of world you are living in. Last August we moved to Japan. We love the big island, the people of Japan and their food. Japan's food is amazing. Max is enjoying the world best tasting fruits and vegetables, abundance of wild fish such as sardines (iwashi), mackerels (saba), herrings (nishin), wagyu-beef, wild sockeye salmon and homemade bouillons (soups, broth) using local ingredients such as organic onions, carrots, broccoli, tomatoes, and my favorite kabocha from the northern island of Hokkaido.

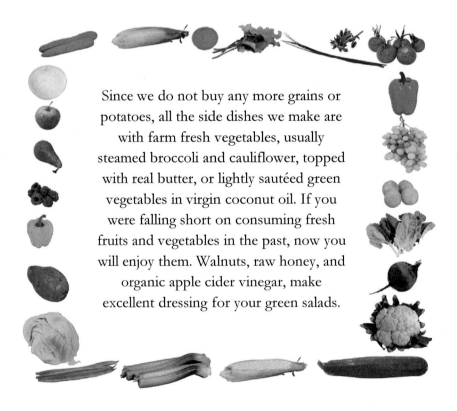

Since we do not buy any more grains or potatoes, all the side dishes we make are with farm fresh vegetables, usually steamed broccoli and cauliflower, topped with real butter, or lightly sautéed green vegetables in virgin coconut oil. If you were falling short on consuming fresh fruits and vegetables in the past, now you will enjoy them. Walnuts, raw honey, and organic apple cider vinegar, make excellent dressing for your green salads.

All the deserts we make at home are made with fruits, nuts, grass-fed butter or virgin coconut oil. We use lots of almond flour, walnut flour, coconut flour for all the cookies and cakes we bake at home twice a week without grains and without sugar.

Almond Flour Belgian Waffle:

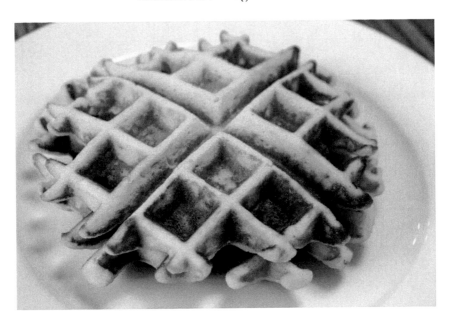

NO GRAIN NO PAIN

Oskar Levsky

oskarlevsky@gmail.com

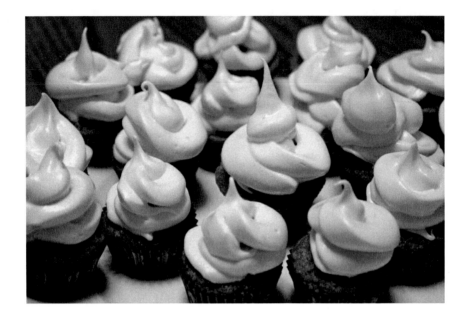

REFERENCES

1. The New England Journal of Medicine 3/17/2005, A Potential Decline in Life Expectancy in the United States, Special Report: http://www.nejm.org/doi/pdf/10.1056/NEJMsr043743

2. American Heart Association, March 18, 2014, Learn and Live, Added Sugars https://www.heart.org/HEARTORG/GettingHealthy/NutritionCenter/HealthyEating/Added-Sugars_UCM_305858_Article.jsp

3. Carolyn McClanahan, 11/28/2011, How Much Should We Spend On Health Care? http://www.forbes.com/sites/carolynmcclanahan/2011/11/28/how-much-should-we-spend-on-health-care-the-big-picture/

4. June 20, 2013 CBS NEWS, Study shows 70 percent of Americans take prescription drugs
http://www.cbsnews.com/news/study-shows-70-percent-of-americans-take-prescription-drugs/

5. Los Angeles Times, November 12, 2013 Written by Melissa Healy About 70 million Americans could take statins under new guidelines
http://articles.latimes.com/2013/nov/12/science/la-sci-sn-statins-cholesterol-new-guidelines-20131112

6. The Weston A. Price Foundation® , Thursday, 24 June, 2004 The Benefits of High Cholesterol, Written by Uffe Ravnskov, MD, PhD
http://www.westonaprice.org/cardiovascular-disease/benefits-of-high-cholesterol

7. Entropy, Volume 15, Issue 4, Pages 1416-1463, Published 18 April 2013 Glyphosate's Suppression of Cytochrome P450 and Amino Acid Biosynthesis by the Gut Microbiome: Pathways to Modern Diseases. Authors: Anthony Samsel and Stephanie Seneff
Text: http://www.mdpi.com/1099-4300/15/4/1416
Video: http://youtu.be/h_AHLDXF5aw

8. "Grain Brain" - The surprising truth about wheat, carbs and sugar – your brain's silent killers by David Perlmutter, MD Published September 17, 2013
http://www.drperlmutter.com/about/grain-brain-by-david-perlmutter/

9. Inflamatory Bowel Disease (IBD), Center For Disease Control and Prevention http://www.cdc.gov/ibd/

10. Inflammatory bowel disease (IBD), Complications, Mayo Clinic
http://www.mayoclinic.org/diseases-conditions/inflammatory-bowel-disease/basics/complications/con-20034908

11. Crohn's Disease, Wikipedia The Free Encyclopedia, 3/26/2014
http://en.wikipedia.org/wiki/Crohn's_disease

12. Excerpt from the book "Challenging Chicago: Coping with Everyday Life, 1837-1920 by Perry Duis (The Risky Business of Food, Milk Wars, Page 135-139) http://www.amazon.com/dp/0252023943/

13. Conjugated linoleic acid content of milk from cows fed different diets. 1999 Oct;82(10):2146-56 US Dairy Forage Research Center USDA, Department of Dairy Science, University of Wisconsin (Dhiman, Anand, Sattler, Pariza) US National Library of Medicine - National Institutes of Health ,
Link: http://www.ncbi.nlm.nih.gov/pubmed/10531600

14. HealthSteward.com
http://www.healthsteward.com/FastFood/KrispyKreme.pdf

15. What's Inside The 26-Ingredient School Lunch Burger?
by Allison Aubrey, Published April 02, 2012 by NPR – National Public Radio
http://www.npr.org/blogs/thesalt/2012/04/02/149717358/whats-inside-the-26-ingredient-school-lunch-burger%20

16. LiveCornFree.com Ingredinets Derived From Corn – What to Avoid, By Sharon Rosen.
http://www.livecornfree.com/2010/04/ingredients-derived-from-corn-what-to.html

17. Food Safety in Canada http://www.hc-sc.gc.ca/fn-an/securit/chem-chim/index-eng.php

18. Linus Pauling Institute Research Report by Regis Moreau, Ph.D LPI Research Associate, Browning: The Dark Side of Sugar
http://lpi.oregonstate.edu/fw04/browning.html

19. Excerpt from the book " The Cure for Heart Disease: Truth Will Save a Nation" by Dwight Lundell, MD ISBN-10 0979034000 Publisher: Heart Surgeons Health Plan; 1st edition (July 10, 2007)
http://amzn.com/0979034000

20. NPR NEWS, How Many Die From Medical Mistakes In U.S. Hospitals? - by Marshall Allen 09/20/2013 http://www.npr.org/blogs/health/2013/09/20/224507654/how-many-die-from-medical-mistakes-in-u-s-hospitals

21. Wednesday, September 26, 2012 by Mike Adams,The Health Ranger http://www.naturalnews.com/037328_russia_gmo_monsanto.html

22. Hippokrates of Kos, (Greek: Ἱπποκράτης; Hippokrátēs; c. 460 – c. 370 BC) Wikipedia – The Free Encyclopedia http://en.wikipedia.org/wiki/Hippocrates

23. Dr. Daniel Rubin, ND, FABNO, Naturopathic Specialists, Scottsdale, Arizona http://www.naturopathicspecialists.com/Oncology.html

24. Sir. Arnold Takemoto, Cancer Control Society, Bioimmune Inc., Scottsdale, Arizona http://www.cancercontrolsociety.com/bio2002/takemoto.html

25. Wikipedia – The Free Encyclopedia, Micotoxins, http://en.wikipedia.org/wiki/Mycotoxin

26. Dr. Michael Gerson "The Second Brain", November 17, 1999 Publisher: Harper Perennia ISBN-10: 0060930721 ISBN-13: 978-0060930721 Link: http://www.amazon.com/The-Second-Brain-Groundbreaking-Understanding/dp/0060930721/ref=pd_sim_b_1?ie=UTF8&refRID=0QHNCGXCFEMPSQ5CATF7

27. GMOs in Food, Institute for Responsible Technology, May 2010 http://www.responsibletechnology.org/gmo-basics/gmos-in-food

28. Journal of Proteomics, Volume 92, October 30, 2013, Pages 248-259 Protein glaciation during aging and in cardiovascular disease http://www.sciencedirect.com/science/article/pii/S1874391913002534

29. Redox Biology, Volume 2, Jaunary 9, 2014, Pages: 411-429
    The role of advanced glycation endproducts in cellular signaling
    http://www.ncbi.nlm.nih.gov/pmc/articles/PMC3949097/

30. Molecular Metabolism Volume 3, Issue 2, April 2014, Pages 94-108
    Vascular effects of advanced glycation end products: Clinical effects
    and molecular mechanisms
    http://www.sciencedirect.com/science/article/pii/S22128778130012
    45

31. Natural News by Mike Adams, The Health Ranger, September 19,
    2012 Eating genetically modified corn (GM corn) and consuming trace
    levels of Monsanto's Roundup chemical fertilizer caused rats to
    develop horrifying tumors, widespread organ damage, and premature
    death. US National Library of Medicine :
    http://www.ncbi.nlm.nih.gov/pmc/articles/PMC2793308/
    http://www.naturalnews.com/037249_gmo_study_cancer_tumors_or
    gan_damage.html

32. Genetic Roulette by Jeffrey Smith http://youtu.be/TB5EBFUwaw0
    Institute for Responsible Technology :
    http://www.responsibletechnology.org

33. The Weston A Price Foundation, How to avoid Genetically Modified
    Foods
    http://www.westonaprice.org/modern-foods/how-to-avoid-gmos

34. Michael Antoniou, Kings College, London School of Medicine,
    9/19/2012 The world's best-selling weed killer, and a genetically
    modified maize resistant to it, can cause tumors, multiple organ
    damage and lead to premature death, a new study has revealed. Link:
    http://www.naturalnews.com/037249_gmo_study_cancer_tumors_or
    gan_damage.html The results of the study were published in The
    Food & Chemistry Toxicology Journal in New York. Read the abstract
    here: http://www.ijbs.com/v05p0706.htm

35. Entropy, Volume 15, Issue 4, Pages 1416-1463, Published 18 April 2013 Glyphosate's Suppression of Cytochrome P450 and Amino Acid Biosynthesis by the Gut Microbiome: Pathways to Modern Diseases. Authors: Anthony Samsel and Stephanie Seneff
Text: http://www.mdpi.com/1099-4300/15/4/1416
Video: http://youtu.be/h_AHLDXF5aw

36. Center for Disease Control and Prevention : "Surgery becomes necessary in Crohn's disease when medications can no longer control the symptoms" http://www.cdc.gov/ibd/

37. Breaking The Vicious Cycle [37] by Elaine Gottschall
http://www.breakingtheviciouscycle.info/

38. Congressman Mike Quigley, November 2010, Reinventing Government, The Federal Budget, Part-1 What is Unsustainable & What We Can Do About it:
http://quigley.house.gov/sites/quigley.house.gov/files/migrated/uploads/quigley_reinventing_government_the_federal_budget_part_1.pdf

39. Andreas Simm - "Protein glycation during aging and in cardiovascular disease " Department of Cardiothoracic Surgery - University Hospital Halle. The research paper was published in a Special Issue of Journal of Proteomics, Volume 92, October 30, 2013, Pages 248-259.
http://www.sciencedirect.com/science/article/pii/S1874391913002534

40. Andreas Simm - "The role of advanced glycation endproducts in cellular signaling". Published in Redox Biology, Volume 2, Jaunary 9, 2014, Pages: 411-429 This research paper is available to the public at http://www.ncbi.nlm.nih.gov/pmc/articles/PMC3949097/

41. "Online Etymology Dictionary." *Online Etymology Dictionary*. N.p., n.d. Web. 25 May 2014.
http://www.etymonline.com/index.php?term=restaurant

42. Cowan, Thomas, MD. "Raw Milk – A Campaign for Real Milk." A Campaign for Real Milk. N.p., 4 Feb. 2014. Web. 25 May 2014. <http://www.realmilk.com/health/raw-milk/

43. Health Benefits of Goat Milk
Ghana Home Page, N.p., n.d. Web. 25 May 2014.
http://www.ghanaweb.com/GhanaHomePage/health/artikel.php?ID=182322

Credits: Teacher Baffour, Cheng S, Lyytikainen A, Kroger H, Lamberg-Allardt C, Alen M, Koistinen A, Wang QJ, Suuriniemi M, Suominen H, Mahonen A, Nicholson PH, Ivaska KK, Korpela R, Ohlsson C, Vaananen KH, Tylavsky F. Effects of calcium, dairy product, and vitamin D supplementation on bone mass accrual and body composition in 10-12-y-old girls: a 2-y randomized trial. Am J Clin Nutr. 2005 Nov;82(5):1115-26. PMID:16280447. Elwood PC, Pickering JE, Fehily AM. Milk and dairy consumption, diabetes and the metabolic syndrome: the Caerphilly prospective study. J Epidemiol Community Health. 2007 Aug;61(8):695-8. PMID:17630368. Ensminger AH, Esminger M. K. J. e. al. Food for Health: A Nutrition Encyclopedia. Clovis, California: Pegus Press; 1986. PMID:15210.

44. Crewe, J.R., MD. "The Milk Cure: Real Milk Cures Many Diseases A Campaign for Real Milk. N.p., Jan. 1929. Web. 25 May 2014. <http://www.realmilk.com/health/milk-cure/

45. "The Maker's Diet": Jordan S. Rubin, Charles F. Stanley: 9781591857143: Amazon.com: Books. N.p., n.d. Web. 25 May 2014. <http://www.amazon.com/Makers-Diet-Jordan-S-Rubin/dp/1591857147

46. Rubin, Jordan. "My Beyond Organic Life | Episode 1 - August 9th." YouTube. YouTube, n.d. Web. 25 May 2014. <https://www.youtube.com/watch?v=tb-wgmni_us&feature=youtu.be

47. Rubin, Jordan. "Beyond Organic." Beyond Organic. N.p., n.d. Web. 25 May 2014. <http://www.mybeyondorganic.com/Products.aspx

48. "Welcome to Organic Pastures." *ORGANIC PASTURES FRESH RAW DAIRY*. N.p., n.d. Web. 25 May 2014. <http://www.organicpastures.com/

49. Garthwaite, Ron, PhD. "Claravale Farm." *Claravale Farm*. N.p., n.d. Web. 25 May 2014. <http://claravaledairy.com/

50. "Raw Goat Milk Benefits." *Raw Goat Milk Benefits*. N.p., n.d. Web. 25 May 2014. <http://www.roseofsharonacres.com/raw_goat_milk_benefits

51. Rural Caprine Farm, Okayama - Japan http://www.yagimilk.com/

52. Gordon, Jeffrey, MD. "Bacterial Bonanza: Microbes Keep Us Alive." *NPR*. NPR, 15 Sept. 2010. Web. 01 June 2014. <http://www.npr.org/templates/story/story.php?storyId=129862107

53. Gordon, Jeffrey MD. "The Gut Response To What We Eat." *NPR*. NPR, 12 Nov. 2009. Web. 01 June 2014. <http://www.npr.org/templates/story/story.php?storyId=120318757

54. Gordon, Jeffrey, MD. "Gut Bacteria May Cause And Fight Disease, Obesity." *NPR*. NPR, 4 Nov. 2008. Web. 01 June 2014. <http://www.npr.org/templates/story/story.php?storyId=95900616

55. Walker, Belinda. *Grain Poisoning of Cattle and Sheep* (n.d.): n. pag. Web. 6 June 2014. <http://www.dpi.nsw.gov.au/__data/assets/pdf_file/0016/101338/grain-poisoning-of-cattle-and-sheep.pdf

56. "Shock Findings in New GMO Study: Rats Fed Lifetime of GM Corn Grow Horrifying Tumors, 70% of Females Die Early." *NaturalNews*. N.p., n.d. Web. 04 June 2014. <http://www.naturalnews.com/037249_gmo_study_cancer_tumors_organ_damage.html

57. Huffstutter, P.J., and Tom Polansek. "Special Report: Lost Hooves, Dead Cattle before Merck Halted Zilmax Sales." *Reuters*. Thomson Reuters, 31 Dec. 2013. Web. 05 June 2014. <http://www.reuters.com/article/2013/12/31/us-zilmax-merck-cattle-special-report-idUSBRE9BT0NV20131231

58. "Smithfield Sale Raises New Questions About the Future of Ractopamine | Food Safety News. "*Food Safety News*. N.p., n.d. Web. 05 June 2014. <http://www.foodsafetynews.com/2013/06/smithfield-sale-raises-new-questions-about-future-of-ractopamine/#.U5BUWf2KCUl

59. "Russia Throws Poisonous Meat Back to US." *English Pravda.ru*. N.p., n.d. Web. 05 June 2014. <http://english.pravda.ru/business/companies/11-12-2012/123129-russia_usa_meat_imports-0/

60. Dr. Mercola, The Secret Sauce in Grass Fed Beef, CLA Benefits Across The Board, N.p., n.d. Web. 5 June 2014. <http://www.mercola.com/beef/cla.htm

61. Over the past 26 years over 400 medical research papers were published about CLA Aydin, Rahim. Conjugated Linoleic Acid: Chemical Structure, Sources and Biological Properties. Turkish Journal of Veterinary & Animal Sciences. 2005;(29):189-195.

62. "Hippocrates."*Wikipedia*. Wikimedia Foundation, 31 May 2014. Web. 04 June 2014. <http://en.wikipedia.org/wiki/Hippocrates

63. Pariza, M. W. "Elsevier." *Elsevier*. N.p., 20 Aug. 1998. Web. 05 June 2014. <http://www.journalofdairyscience.org/article/S0022-0302%2899%2975458-5/abstract

64. "Meat."*NZTE*. N.p., n.d. Web. 05 June 2014. <https://www.nzte.govt.nz/en/buy/our-sectors/food-and-beverage/meat/

65. "Kobe Beef."*Wikipedia*. Wikimedia Foundation, 06 Mar. 2014. Web. 05 June 2014. <http://en.wikipedia.org/wiki/Kobe_beef

66. Takada, Aya. "Japanese Farmers Bet on Steaks Costing Twice the Price of Silver."*Bloomberg.com*. Bloomberg, 3 Apr. 2014. Web. 06 June 2014. <http://www.bloomberg.com/news/2014-04-03/japan-clothing-cattle-to-spur-pricey-wagyu-steak-exports.html

67. "Japanese Cuisine Wins Cultural Heritage Status."*The Japan Times - News RSS*. N.p., 5 Dec. 2013. Web. 06 June 2014. <http://www.japantimes.co.jp/news/2013/12/05/national/japanese-cuisine-added-to-unesco-intangible-heritage-list/#.U5FM0_2KCUn

68. Tsubota-Utsugi, Megumi. "Diets High in Animal Protein May Help Prevent Functional Decline in Elderly Individuals." *ScienceDaily*. ScienceDaily, 11 Mar. 2014. http://www.sciencedaily.com/releases/2014/03/140311163101.htm#.U3tTSFIrIUg.blogger

69. Dr. Mercola, "Top 10 Ways the American Health Care System Fails."*Mercola.com*. N.p., 15 Mar. 2014. Web. 06 June 2014. <http://articles.mercola.com/sites/articles/archive/2014/03/15/bad-american-health-care-system.aspx

70. Dr. Mercola, "10 Common US Foods That Are Banned in Other Countries."*Mercola.com*. N.p., 10 July 2013. Web. 06 June 2014. <http://articles.mercola.com/sites/articles/archive/2013/07/10/banned-foods.aspx

71. "Bible Gateway Passage: Leviticus 11:9-12 - American Standard Version." *Bible Gateway*. N.p., n.d. Web. 06 June 2014. <http://www.biblegateway.com/passage/?search=Leviticus+11%3A9-12&version=ASV

72. Weissmann, M.D., Gerald, M.D. "Scientists Show How DHA Resolves Inflammation." *ScienceDaily*. ScienceDaily, 1 July 2013. Web. 07 June 2014.

<http://www.sciencedaily.com/releases/2013/07/130701135442.htm

73. Ryal, Julian. "World's Oldest Person Celebrates Her 116th Birthday: 'Eat and Sleep and You Will Live a Long Time'" *The Telegraph*. Telegraph Media Group, 2 Mar. 2014. Web. 07 June 2014. <http://www.telegraph.co.uk/news/worldnews/asia/japan/1067046 7/Worlds-oldest-person-celebrates-her-116th-birthday-Eat-and-sleep-and-you-will-live-a-long-time.html

74. "Herring Season" الشرق لصحيفة محفوظة الحقوق جميع - الرنجة موسم This Article Was Published in Asharq Al-printed No. (564) Page (24) on 20/06/2013 Middle Newspaper 20/06/2013 http://www.alsharq.net.sa/contact <http://www.alsharq.net.sa/2013/06/20/872465

75. Macedonia – Timeless, *EM*. N.p., n.d. Web. 05 June 2014. <http://www.exploringmacedonia.com/

76. John Wood, U.S. Wellness Meats, The Grassfed Difference. http://youtu.be/ae-BaOGVpJY

77. Dr. Mercola Discusses Turkeys and Beef with Joel Salatin at Polyface Farm http://youtu.be/UXOtq2J-mNk

78. Jordan Rubin, My Beyond Organic Life, Episode-1, August 9th http://youtu.be/tb-wgmni_us

79. Jordan Rubin, "Journey from Sickness to Health" http://youtu.be/fjNCGx8fc0w

80. Seneff, Stephanie. "Stephanie Seneff on Sulfur (Interview)."*Mercola.com*. N.p., 17 Sept. 2011. Web. 13 June 2014. <http://articles.mercola.com/sites/articles/archive/2011/09/17/step hanie-seneff-on-sulfur.aspx>

81. "Scientists Show How DHA Resolves Inflammation."*ScienceDaily*. ScienceDaily, n.d. Web. 13 June 2014. <http://www.sciencedaily.com/releases/2013/07/130701135442.htm>.

82. "Health Benefits of Conjugated Linoleic Acid."*Mercola.com*. N.p., n.d. Web. 13 June 2014. <http://www.mercola.com/beef/cla.htm>

83. Stirban, Alin, Thomas Gawlowski, and Michael Roden. "Vascular Effects of Advanced Glycation Endproducts; Clinical Effects and Molecular Mechanism." *Elsevier : Article Locator*. Molecular Metabolism Volume 3, Issue 2, April 2014, Pages 94–108, n.d. Web. 20 June 2014. http://www.sciencedirect.com/science/article/pii/S2212877813001245

84. Primal Defense, Ultimate Probiotic Formula http://www.gardenoflife.com/Products-for-Life/Digestive-Health/Primal-Defense-ULTRA.aspx

Made in the USA
San Bernardino, CA
29 February 2016